BEN KAPLAN

FEET, DON'T FAIL ME NOW

THE ROGUE'S GUIDE TO RUNNING THE MARATHON

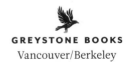

GREYSTONE BOOKS

Vancouver/Berkeley

Greystone Books Ltd.
www.greystonebooks.com

Cataloguing data available from Library and Archives Canada
ISBN 978-1-77100-073-4 (pbk.)
ISBN 978-1-77100-074-1 (epub)

Editing by Nancy Flight
Copy editing by Lucy Kenward
Cover design by Peter Cocking and Jessica Sullivan
Interior design by Jessica Sullivan
Cover photograph by iStockphoto.com
Printed and bound in Canada by Friesens
Distributed in the U.S. by Publishers Group West

We gratefully acknowledge the financial support of the Canada Council for the Arts, the British Columbia Arts Council, the Province of British Columbia through the Book Publishing Tax Credit, and the Government of Canada through the Canada Book Fund for our publishing activities.

Greystone Books is committed to reducing the consumption of old-growth forests in the books it publishes. This book is one step toward that goal.

For Julie, magic Julie, who wanted to wear a
shirt that said, "Enough, already, about running,"
at the Boston Marathon. You're rock 'n' roll.

CONTENTS

A NOTE TO
THE RUNNER

USING THIS book, you're going to get to the marathon in a year by completing four races: the 5K, 10K, half-marathon, and marathon. It will be difficult—fun, but difficult—but I know it can be done because I did it. And I started four months before my wife, Julie, and I were expecting our first kid.

I've run six marathons, two 30Ks, four half-marathons, and three 10Ks. Plenty of people have run more and run faster, but that's why I'm a good tour guide: I'm average, and the bar that I set isn't really that high. As a reporter for Canada's *National Post* newspaper, I've spent the past five years covering running, gathering tips, testing out sneakers, speaking with experts, and, every once in awhile, running a race.

The workout plan set forth here isn't mine—it's the experts': Dr. James Pivarnik, director of the Center for Physical Activity and Health at Michigan State University; Dave Scott-Thomas, head coach of the Speed River Track and Field Club in Guelph, Ontario, who trains two out of three Canadian Olympic marathon runners; Seanna Robinson, founder of the resource blog RunningWell; Dr. Ralph Vernacchia, co-chair of the USA Track & Field Sport Psychology Sub-committee and director of the Center for Performance Excellence at Western Washington University; Matt Loiselle, competitive Canadian marathon runner; and Josphat Nzinga, a Kenyan racer who trained with the world's fastest people and whose uncle won Boston three times. All I do is ask questions, experiment with the answers, and write down what works. To get to the marathon, in essence, run a little, then some more, then keep running until you can go 42.2K (26.2 miles). But first, a few steps before you begin:

STEP 1: Choose four races—5K, 10K, half-marathon, and marathon—spread out, in that order, over a year, with a new race about every three months. For now, maybe just sign up for the first two. Who knows? You might meet some new people and want to run with them at a race somewhere interesting.

STEP 2: Begin the week-by-week training program, in which you work up to a new race distance every thirteen weeks. At the end of each section, I document my event for that segment to give you a sense of what to expect on the road. Now, my races won't correspond with yours exactly. I'm trying to qualify for Boston, and so I need to first run a marathon in 3:10. This will be my second race, which is when you run 10K. But whether it's a marathon or a jog around the block, we're all doing the same thing—going as fast as we can and keeping going, even when we get tired. Your races might be spaced out differently; that's also fine. Each chapter contains a note called "The Finish Line," which gives you workouts based on how far you are from your race. No one run will get you to the marathon, and no one day—whether it's hill repeats, a long run, or a speed workout—will make you faster. It's about the gradual accumulation of mileage. If you have extra time between races, repeat a week of the program. If you have less time, don't skip a run.

STEP 3: Get a calendar and mark it up as you train. Record how fast and how far you run, what you eat, how you're feeling. You're about to embark on a journey. Keep a logbook of how far you go.

STEP 4: Enjoy the process. Remember, you're not getting paid or competing for your country, and, when you're running with 45,000 people, you're probably not going to win. The average woman takes almost five hours to complete the marathon and the average dude around four and a quarter—an awful lot of time to be doing anything, an impossible amount of time to be doing something you despise.

STEP 5: Pick your starting point. The program's designed to be followed week by week, but not everyone's starting at the same place. If you're not sure what distance you should be running, try the workouts in Chapters 2, 8, 15, or 21, which is where each distance's training really kicks in. By beginning in the middle of the program you'll miss some stories, advice, and great music, but you'll find a race-specific workout for whatever distance you choose.

STEP 6: Customize your own workout. The ones in the book are guidelines, not commandments. Different people will be able to do different things. I'm writing this book thinking cautiously about Julie, who's thirty-five, sporty, and just had a kid. While the program works with basic principles—long slow runs, speed work, cross-training, maintenance jogs, and hill workouts—the number of repetitions, the time spent running and walking, and the intensity level can be modified.

STEP 7: Load up your iPod. Costas Karageorghis, sports psychologist with London's Brunel University School of Sport and Education, says, "Music has the propensity to enhance how we feel, even at high-exercise intensity" and adds that music reduces the perception of effort by 10 percent, can increase endurance by 9 percent, and provides a 15 percent boost in motivation. "Music predisposes us to want to work out. Music that's arousing functions like a stimulant or legal drug."

To that end, each chapter features a custom-made running set list, designed by some of the world's biggest artists (and some I just love). Perhaps some of the tunes will have the same beats per minute as your running heart rate and stride—something fast, in the 130 to 170 beats-per-minute range, like Daft Punk's "Get Lucky," "Jumpin' Jack Flash" by The Rolling Stones, and "Jai Ho," the theme song from the movie *Slumdog Millionaire*—but what's more important is to run to music you like. The musicians aren't necessarily runners—but we're not asking them for advice about sneakers, we're assembling a collection of awesome songs.

STEP 8: Talk to your doctor before you begin. Not just if you're old or if you have heart trouble, but everyone. People die at races. This program is about improving, not risking, your life.

FINALLY: This is your book and it's a rogue's guide. Start wherever, read whatever, skip whenever, run however. It's not a textbook, it's an outline and a motivational screed. Use it any way you want . . . just don't forget to lace up your shoes.

ONE

ENTERING THE GREAT UNKNOWN

ON THE ROAD TO 5K

"I'm a lazy son of a bitch, I can't lie."

WOODY HARRELSON, a runner, on why it took him twenty-eight years to complete *Bullet for Adolf*, his autobiographical play

LET'S GET
IT STARTED

THE TRAINING: Cementing a Schedule that Works

WEEK 1: Twice, walk outside for 20 minutes. On your return, run when you can see your home. If the first walk is easy, on the second, jog for 4 minutes, 10 minutes into your walk.

WEEK 2: Twice, walk and jog for 25 minutes. At each 5-minute interval, jog for 60 seconds. If this feels easy, play with the proportions. The important thing is twice-a-week consistency.

THE SOUNDTRACK: will.i.am

THE FINISH LINE: The 5K, now just about 13 weeks away.

START RUNNING right now in whatever clothes you have. Pick two days this week and make a commitment to go outside and walk for twenty minutes. Don't even start running until you've been out for eighteen minutes, are on your way home, and can see your house. Do that once, and you've crossed a threshold. Do it twice, taking a day off in between, and you'll build momentum. Next week, start again. Jog for one minute every five. This part—getting out the door and adding more running—is hard, but it's also awesome. At no point will you improve more quickly than when you begin.

You don't need fancy shoes or yellow underpants. You don't need a trainer, a quinoa diet, a $500 watch, a Kenyan passport, or, for that matter, a medium-sized waist. What you do need to do is decide why you're running. If you're going to squeeze in a run before work or after you put the kids to bed, if you're going to stick with this program for an entire year, if you're going to pay money to participate in an activity that's going to hurt—it's good to know what you're doing it for. Is it to lose weight, to challenge yourself, to change? Once you've figured out why you're running, keep this motivation in your sneakers because it's a long, time-consuming road from the couch to the marathon. And it's quite possible your nipples will bleed from chafing during the distance runs along the way. (Two fingers' worth of petroleum jelly and a decent T-shirt will prevent that, but the point is: running ain't always going to be margaritas aboard Jimmy Buffett's Barefoot Islands cruise.)

The thing is, running is something we've evolved for. Human evolutionary biologist Dr. Daniel Lieberman is so famous for his work at Harvard University that he doesn't take appointments to talk to the press. If he did, he says, he wouldn't have time to do his work. You just have to call the guy and get lucky. So one afternoon, I pick up the phone.

"Largely because nobody had worked on the subject, we took our time, and, indeed, I think made the case that human beings have evolved to run long distances," says Lieberman, whose research in human physiology—the way we breathe, the way our head sits on our necks, the way we've evolved with less hair and longer heels than other primates—points to a prehistoric survival technique known as "persistence hunting."

Before ancient man had bows and arrows or knew how to carve stones into knives, our forebears used to run down their dinner or risk becoming dinner themselves. We've survived, chasing down antelope and saber-toothed tigers, like Chris McDougall's book of the same name says, because we're "born to run." When our ancestors evolved from the monkeys, Lieberman believes our bodies adapted so we could kill our prey by chasing it, either until it died of heat exhaustion or until it was so worn out from all that running that it was an easy mark, ready to be cooked over a flame.

"Putting a stone point on a spear to make it lethal was invented less than 300,000 years ago, but man has been eating meat for two-and-a-half million years. How'd they do it?" asks Lieberman, a long-distance runner who recently completed his first Boston Marathon. "It's no fluke why we look the way that we do. Running is part of our basic biology, and when people say that it's strange to run marathon distances, that's farcical. That's what mankind has evolved to do."

Lieberman sometimes works with Campbell Rolian, an anatomy postdoctoral fellow at the University of Calgary. Rolian tested the amount of muscle force generated by our toes in both walking and running and produced evidence that our toes reduce injury and save energy while we run. Our toes don't do anything for us when we walk.

"By having shorter toes, you can achieve significant energy savings when running, energy which could then be used to reproduce," says Rolian, also a runner, making the point that only the best long-distance runners survived long enough to pass on their genes. You either ran or you died, so the cavemen who lived—your forefathers—had to be fast. Genetically, you're sprung from the greatest runners of all time.

IN 2012, twelve million Americans paid to cross some kind of finish line, and for the first time in history, more than half of those participants were women. In Canada, more than one million people own running shoes. That's one in thirty-three, which is pretty good considering half the country is covered in snow. Races can't keep up with demand: the 2013 Berlin Marathon sold out 40,000 places in three-and-a-half hours, while all 45,000 entries to the 2012 Chicago Marathon sold out in six days—three weeks faster than in 2011. Eighty-five thousand people bought tickets for either $65 or $80 (depending on when they registered) to participate in 2013's City2Surf run in Sydney, Australia—and plenty were turned away. Think about that: there are more people who want to pay to go jogging at 8 a.m. than there are spots for them at the starting line.

Why are so many freaking people running, and why are they all freaking doing it right freaking now? Because races got shorter, women got their own sneakers, and running clinics have taken over the world. Today, jogging classes are everywhere—from Lahore, Pakistan, to downtown Milwaukee, to the Al Asad Airbase west of Baghdad in Iraq. In Canada, some 800,000 people have attended a Running Room clinic, which costs $70, meets three times a week for up to four months, and trains people to run. Thirty years ago, the place didn't exist, and now two-thirds of the customers who buy a pair of sneakers at the Running Room also take one of their courses. Even just a decade ago, people would have laughed at the idea of someone teaching you how to run. "What can they tell you?" they'd have said. "Don't run into that tree?!"

I laughed too, then I led a class at the Running Room and stopped laughing, because the clinics work. Mostly it's just because we get folks out and running. It's easier to run when you form a social group, have a goal, and are surrounded by good-looking strangers who provide accountability and support. We give runners a program, a time, a place to go. This is what I aim to reproduce here: a sense of community; a series of goals, tips, and reasons to believe in yourself. Have you ever taken a good look at a runner? Let me tell you, we don't all look like Carl Lewis. As often as not, we look like the people at the food court in the local mall.

"I thought, Who am I to be running? I'm just a regular, everyday person with padding. Running's for super-thin people—like, Kenyan-thin—not for people like me," says Lesley Taylor, who was so shy when she began running that she'd only use her office treadmill on Saturday mornings, when no one was there. "I had a vision in my head of what a runner looks like, and I wasn't it." Taylor, a casual smoker whose weight had crept up to more than 220 pounds as she approached her fifties, had finally had enough of her lifestyle and decided to change. At first, she began setting tiny, achievable goals for herself on her Saturday morning pilgrimages. "I remember being on the treadmill and reading something in *Cosmo*—and that's how slow I was going, I was able to read—and it said the first ten to fifteen minutes are the hardest. I thought, Ten to fifteen minutes? Are you nuts?!"

But Taylor entered a 5K (3 miles) with some friends from her office and surprised herself with how well she did. She didn't win. She *survived*. And then she got off the treadmill and started running outside. This is important. This week, if you do nothing else, get outside. Taylor was embarrassed when she started—we all are—but she did it, and it's the single most important step you can take, because you're going to have to enter some races to become a runner, and you'll be hard-pressed to find one that takes place in a gym. "I felt like I stuck out like a sore thumb," Taylor says, "but I did it again, and then I did it again, and soon I realized that people weren't really looking at me. They probably have their own stuff going on."

After her 5K, Taylor followed a friend's lead to a running clinic for a 10K (6-mile) race. She just wanted to see if she could go that distance. Soon, she found herself making new friends. "It became a social thing," Taylor says, adding that she began to make lifestyle decisions to better serve her new hobby. Like a lot of us, she still likes her wine, but as she became buddies with her running partners, she cut out the casual ciggie—none of her new friends smoked—and early-morning runs on the weekend slowly replaced after-work drinks.

"It's not like I ever sat down and decided: I'm going to become a runner," she says. "Gradually, things just started to change." This is how you get to the marathon. It doesn't happen overnight. But you don't have to be a college athlete, a monk, or a vegan. You don't have to be skinny, live beside a cornfield, or hire a nanny to take care of your kids. You don't have to get a Reebok tattooed on your ass.

RIGHT NOW, sign up for a race. It's too easy to skip a day when nothing's at stake. Find a 5K close to home—there are more than five thousand races in North America each year—and register for the one that's three months away. You may just be starting out but, over time, over a year, you'll improve. You'll run farther. Run faster. Feel yourself getting quicker, your body parts working in harmony, and instead of dreading your workouts you'll actually feel excited about your next run.

Buy a calendar and use it as a logbook. Circle your race dates. On your training days, write down how long you ran, how far, and how you felt during and after the run. Keep track of your progress. A record of your accomplishments can be reassuring come race day. Running provides positive affirmations. Each time you do something you've never done before, you cross a new threshold. Write it down. When you see yourself increasing your mileage, you'll want to increase it some more. Because a 5K run is a challenge. It can mean running for more than an hour. That's why it's imperative that you keep up with the training, especially when you're just getting started.

So figure out a schedule you can commit to, and skip the hamburger on the way home from work. Pump your arms a bit and pick up your feet when you walk. Lift your knees and try to keep your back straight. Tilt your head back slightly and remember to breathe. We'll learn all about form and technique later, as well as the latest electronic doo-dads and duds, but for now, just walk swiftly. Pretend your bus is about to leave.

Running is fun, healthy, and cheap, and it's a great way of exploring where you live. It opens your mind and makes you feel good, forces you to take a break from the rat race, and gets you out of the house. Running changes your mood.

It's not genes or sneakers or a fancy track program that will get you to the marathon. It's just doing it again and again and again. Time commitments are going to be a challenge, but the time you spend running will help prepare you for the moments that matter: the ones when you need to stand still.

THE SOUNDTRACK: will.i.am
will.i.am is a tough guy to get a bead on; for instance, I never know how to punctuate his name, and his album title includes a hashtag. In person, he's soft-spoken and laid-back—possibly stoned—and seems to lose track of my questions as if I'm speaking in Hebrew. Then, out of nowhere, like Will Ferrell in the debate scene in *Old School,* he provides an insightful response.

I tell him "Let's Get It Started" has been called the best running song of all time and he's silent, then inspired, as if taking instruction from above: "It has a lot of tempo blocks and changes, accelerations, and it speeds, but isn't too speedy— it's the pace of a jog you can do for a long time," he says. He adds that after "Let's Get It Started" was co-opted in sporting arenas, it changed the way he wrote music for The Black Eyed Peas. (The group's next record, *The E.N.D.*, sold eleven million copies and was nominated for six Grammy Awards.)

"You can't run to the pace of electro music for a long time, but you can run to "Let's Get It Started" for an hour; it's 95 beats per minute, an endurance beat, marathon pace," he says. "One hundred and thirty beats per minute isn't a sprint, but it's a fast run, and 142 beats per minute is like hard house; that's damn near a sprint. Those motherfuckers are on speed."

When recommending his own running songs, will.i.am gets sentimental, going back to the music of his childhood and suggesting tunes based not on BPMS but on a feeling he gets when he listens to early hip hop. This is important. When you are programming music, it doesn't matter how fast a song is. What matters is how the song makes you feel.

"Jenifa Taught Me (Derwin's Revenge)," De La Soul: "That was my world. The beats were nuts and the words [here he starts rapping]: *The Downstairs/where we met/I'd brought records/ she'd cassettes. 3 Feet High and Rising* changed everything. I was fourteen years old, and that still gets me going today."

"My Philosophy," Boogie Down Productions: "To this day, KRS-One is one of my favorite rappers. *You got to have style/ and learn to be original.* That sentence influenced me. The song's not extra-fast, but you can work out to it and not get too, too tired, but have a healthy workout, sweat."

2

EVERYTHING
SNEAKERS

THE TRAINING: Introducing a Third Run

WEEK 3: Jog and walk for 25 minutes twice this week, trying to increase the proportion of jogging to walking time.

WEEK 4: Do last week's workout, but try to build on its proportions. For instance, with every 5-minute interval, try to run 2 minutes, walk 1, then run 2. Try that 5 times and record the results in your logbook.

WEEK 5: Work in a third day and stretch all your workouts to 30 minutes. Maybe you can run for 5 minutes and walk for 1 all the way up to 30? Maybe not. Experiment. Play.

THE SOUNDTRACK: Paul Simon

THE FINISH LINE: The 5K, now just about 11 weeks away.

AFTER SPENDING two weeks outside running and walking for twenty minutes each time, bump up your workouts to twenty-five minutes and aim to increase the amount of time you run. Wear a watch (any watch) and fill out your logbook.

Always open your workouts with a few minutes of walking, but then get funky. At five minutes, run for a minute. Then try it again at ten. At twelve-and-a-half minutes, when you head for home, run again. Go slowly, but see how long your jog can last. Feel free. On each run, try to break your last run's record and embrace that idea: You're not just walking around your neighborhood, you're preparing for a race. You're not just walking in circles—you're training for the marathon!

By Week 5, aim to introduce a third run into your schedule and, as time permits, take a day off between workouts. Again, the proportion of running to walking isn't really what we're after: the goal is to keep to your schedule, maintain a logbook, and commit to the long haul. *Rome*, the fantastic record by Danger Mouse featuring Jack White and Norah Jones, wasn't built in a day.

At the Running Room, workouts start with walking for ten minutes and then running for one, but you know your own capabilities. The trick is to write everything down, and keep the workouts varied. Even if the difference is as subtle as just walking a little bit faster, no two runs should be identical from week to week. They're also getting longer. By the end of Week 5, you'll have spent thirty minutes outside, three times. If you're conscious of the training, understand that each workout is building the foundation for what's next. How can running be boring when it changes each day?

When you're out there, give yourself challenges. Run to the next mailbox or, in my neighborhood, the Portuguese chicken joint. Remember, this is playtime. It's OK to be goofy. Ben Errett, my running partner and friend, sometimes sings Carly Rae Jepsen while racing. I like that running is my time to be a kid, to go out in a rainstorm, to yell. Do whatever it takes to keep yourself motivated and happy. Once you've run for a while, watch how it becomes addictive and spreads. Never mind the escalator, you'll say. I'll take the stairs. Of course, plenty of people would rather be dragged 5K by their eyelids than pay to run that far in a race. And often I wish that instead of running past that chicken place, I were stopping in for six wings and a beer. That's fine. Running is not always a pool party and your habits aren't going to change overnight. It's possible that you won't even like running, which is why you should run a few times before buying shoes. On your run this evening, if you hope that each passing car hits you, perhaps you should try rollerblading instead. However, if that sensation—or a car—doesn't strike you and you're ready to commit to your goal, it's time to go get some shoes.

RUNNING SHOES are made out of leather and rubber and work best when they're worn on your feet. The first ones were created by Charles Goodyear (who, ironically, will forever be associated with cars), and they're often made in Indonesia, China, and Vietnam. They consist of a sole and an upper, the part that cradles your foot, and have a layer of foam between the two to cushion your foot and provide support, especially in the heel.

No doubt you've heard about "barefoot running," which is usually done in sneakers, just models with little foam or other materials between your foot and the ground. They're designed to protect your feet from abrasion without inhibiting natural motion. Minimal shoes are like barefoot shoes but they provide more cushioning for runners who need more support than a barefoot shoe gives but still want their feet to roll and flex as if they weren't wearing shoes at all. Traditional running shoes provide even more cushioning and, depending on the model, varying levels of support for the feet. It's generally accepted that most people pronate to a degree—that it's a natural part of our walking and running motion—but also that "stability" and "motion control" shoes designed to prevent the foot from rolling too far inward or outward may have altered people's natural running stride.

No one's truly certain, but the emphasis now is on reducing the "drop" between a running shoe's heel and toe height to encourage a more natural gait. While it's still possible to buy heavily padded and posted running shoes, the trend is toward minimal drop (4mm to 8mm in so-called transition shoes) and zero-drop shoes. It all seems really complicated but really it isn't. Sneaker companies, masters of obfuscation, are always coming up with the next new thing. Science then usually refutes it. If the shoe fits, wear it—that's my expert advice.

When you go to buy shoes, go in the afternoon rather than in the morning, as feet swell during the bump and grind of the typical day. On a long run, feet can swell a whole shoe size, so your sneakers are the one piece of running gear that you don't want to fit too snugly. Also, if you lose weight with this program, don't be surprised if you go down a shoe size. It happens. Write it down.

"When I started running, I went and got a random pair of shoes, and my feet pretty much always hurt," says Samantha Danbert, a graduate student in exercise physiology at Michigan State. Danbert thought she had developed a stress fracture, a tiny crack in the bone, and went to see her doctor. Also an athlete, her doctor recommended a visit to Runners, a sneaker specialty shop in Saginaw, Michigan. "When you go into Runners, they have lanes like on a track and they watch you walk without shoes to determine what kind of sneakers you need," Danbert says. In an ideal foot strike, runners first land on the balls of the foot, moving a little laterally to absorb the landing and then rolling through the foot with each footfall. When we run, our feet hit the ground like a wave breaking across the beach; the foot lands, rolls, lifts, and then repeats the process again and again. We all do this differently. With a good pair of sneakers, the only shock you should feel is their sticker price.

"I thought I hated running, but what I really hated was running in the wrong shoes. I tend to run on the outside of my foot, I don't overpronate, but my sneakers get worn down after about three months because of the way I land," says Danbert, who is training for the Olympic Trials as we speak. "Everything changed with my relationship to the sport when I started wearing the right shoes."

SNEAKER SALES in the United States reached nearly $10 billion last year, and more than a quarter of athletic shoes sold are specifically designed for running. They're worn by Pippa Middleton, *MasterChef*'s Joe Bastianich, and Usain Bolt. They're light. When I stopped wearing my dad's old shoes and was sent some proper sneakers, it felt like stepping into a cloud. They made me want to run, and run quickly. However, just because a publicly traded company says that a barefoot shoe will make you so fast you can chase down a gazelle or that a gait-correcting sneaker with a cushioned heel the size of a Pygmy will save your knees doesn't necessarily make that so.

A Swiss former high school track star, Benno Nigg is the founder of the Human Performance Lab in Calgary and has spent thirty years studying running biomechanics, which makes him a bit of an expert in feet. Adidas and Reebok have hired him to help design sneakers that will keep runners from getting hurt. "There are quite a few studies, but the results don't always point in the same direction," Nigg says. Sneakers might help you, he told me, but they also might not.

"Everybody wants to correct pronation. I've been studying this for three decades, and at the beginning I thought that pronation was dangerous and that we have to reduce it, but then when I went deeper I realized that's not the case." Today, Nigg believes that pronation is the natural movement of the foot as it lands. The foot can fall in one of three ways and, not surprisingly, there's a sneaker for each: neutral (which actually means up to 15 degrees of inward roll), overpronated (more than 15 degrees of inward roll), or supinated (outward roll). "There's nothing wrong with pronation," Nigg says. "I don't think there needs to be a correction to overpronation in most cases."

Researcher Michael Ryan also asks you not to overthink shoes. "I've become increasingly suspicious of these specialized shoes, motion-control shoes, pronation-correcting shoes, and think we should give everyday runners a little more credit," says Ryan, who makes the point that injuries haven't decreased and times haven't gotten any faster since the advent of high-tech modern footwear. In his 2010 paper for the *British Journal of Sports Medicine*, Ryan assembled eighty-one female runners, looked at how their feet hit the ground when they run, and divided the runners into pronators, overpronators, and those with a neutral stride. He then matched up the runners with the shoes that were designed for their feet and gait and recorded any injuries they sustained while running.

Form-correcting sneakers are not an exact science, and Ryan's results were startling. Even after he tested how his subjects landed and matched them with appropriate footwear, the runners were no less likely to stave off injury or improve their performance than if they had selected their sneakers at random. Samantha Danbert's experience did not match up with what Ryan discovered in his lab.

"It's become popular for people to feel like they're under-supported, but when we put all these people in sneakers marketed with a 'technical edge,' shoes with either greater heel or more cushioning at the toe, depending on what the shoe companies would have you believe, we found that they don't prevent injury. A lot of assumptions were not supported by facts," Ryan says. According to his study, which had the women all complete a thirteen-week half-marathon training program in their specialized shoes, participants in the motion-controlled sneakers—the ones that were designed to help runners who overpronate—reported the most missed training days due to injury.

"If you're new to running, it hurts, and training comes down to a runner knowing their body—when to increase the workload and when to back off," says Ryan. "Modern sneakers are terrific, but I wouldn't expect them to do all the work."

When I ask Nigg how he would advise my mother-in-law to pick out sneakers, his answer's simple: "If the shoe is comfortable, that seems to be an indication that the forces are right," he says. "If it doesn't feel right, it's probably not the right shoe."

THE MOST POPULAR running shoes sold last year in North America were the Nike Free series, which is designed for neutral runners. I'm a neutral runner and you probably are, too. According to Reed Ferber, director of the Running Injury Clinic in Calgary, 85 percent of runners land with a neutral footfall. Of course, if you're among the other 15 percent, that statistic doesn't mean much. Just know that you probably aren't.

When you head to the store to try on sneakers, take in the ones you've been wearing. The salesperson may be able to tell from the wear pattern how your feet strike the ground.

Remember, sneakers aren't automobiles. There's nothing hidden under the hood. And they aren't baseball mitts. They don't have to be broken in. Before you buy anything, a store should let you sample its product. Take a spin around the block or go for a jog on an instore treadmill. Get to know what you're buying and like it, or else shop around.

The shoes you buy now may or may not be the ones you wear to your marathon a year from now. It depends on how cheap you are. Generally, sneakers last about five months or 550 kilometers (roughly 350 miles), but you'll know when your footwear needs a spruce-up. It might be when you need a psychological boost or when you feel like you're developing an injury. I change sneakers a lot, but that's because I write about them for the newspaper and haven't had to buy a pair since dumping my dad's old trainers in the trash. I've run in Nike, New Balance, Brooks, Asics, Mizuno, Saucony, and Adidas— basically any brand someone sends me—and I've found they all work pretty well. We're not running through fire, across water, or over broken glass. There's no "best" sneaker. It's all just a matter of sale price and choice. Again, what you like— what you'll wear—is the best shoe for you: leave your shoes in the closet and they won't do a lick of good.

When I went shopping for sneakers, I brought an Olympic track coach and a fashion designer with me. Barrie Shepley coached Canada's Olympic triathletes to gold in 2000. A former track star, Shepley's whole life is shoes. So it's funny to hear him dis the goods.

"Most of this stuff's similar because the big companies steal each other's technology," Shepley says, echoing what I heard from the guy who designs for Timex, that in his business of GPS watches all the major companies use the same hardware. The Timex guy actually joked that while at least the watch companies use different manufacturers (that all do the same thing), different brands of shoes are sometimes made in the same factories overseas. "There's no reason a beginner runner needs to spend more than a hundred bucks on sneakers," continues Shepley, "none of them are going to help you if you don't wear them anyways."

So let's say that you're going to pick out your shoes based entirely on comfort. You've been correctly wearing footwear since you were fifteen months old, and your feet have been OK until now. Let's just assume this trend will continue as you train for your 5K. Then the next question is: How do they look?

Shawn Hewson is the creative director of the sportswear label Bustle Clothing, and he's probably the first customer to shop for sneakers at the Running Room wearing Prada from sunglasses to socks. Hewson's a judge on *Project Runway Canada*, and he wishes running shoes would turn down the lights. "A lot of this stuff's like, 'Hey, look at me, I'm a runner!'" says Hewson, adding that when it comes to sportswear, whether shopping for the slopes or the pool, when you're just getting started, neutral colors are the best bet. "All I know is that if I see someone in fluorescent yellow sneakers, they better be pretty fast."

To make runners feel fast, sneaker companies have come up with a more-is-more approach to shoe design. On many a pair, you've got squiggles, circles, stripes, and squares; reds, yellow, greens, and blues; raised heels, exaggerated toes, bright yellow laces, fluorescent tongues... all on the same poor pair of kicks. Hewson sees nothing wrong with plain black: "I thought shoes would look sleeker today than when I used to run, but they've gotten uglier," he says. "You want something that looks clean and functional, elegant and sexy, like a race car that sits on the starting line."

Your running shoes are an opportunity to pick out that sports car that you can't get in real life. Choose a pair that makes you excited, that makes you feel confident, that makes you want to run. Sneakers will help alleviate the force of impact, and the right pair will give you a mental edge. Enjoy the process and make yourself happy, but the right shoes will not get rid of the work behind this week's twenty-five-minute walk-runs.

Heart will. Kathrine Switzer, the first woman to register for and complete the Boston Marathon, took a razor blade to her $26 Adidas sneakers in 1967 because the webbing was pinching her toes. She not only finished that race but dodged a race official to do so. And the late Danny Kassap, a long-distance runner originally from Congo, wore his buddy's wife's sneakers while competing in the Canadian 10K Road Race Championships in 2002, a race he won. And I love the story about the Kenyan runners Gilbert Kiptoo and Luka Chelimo. Kiptoo won a race in Thunder Bay and earned $2,000, a fortune back home in Kenya, and so he gave Chelimo his old shoes. Chelimo then wore those shoes to compete in an Australian marathon—which, like Kiptoo, he won. Don't overthink shoes.

Eleven weeks out from your first 5K, hopefully you're getting the hang of this training. Are you sleeping better? Missing last call? Bothering your friends with running updates on Facebook? Stretching by the copy machine? You're now running three times a week and should be doubling the proportion of minutes spent running to walking. Write it all down, and please, never, ever, pay retail for shoes.

THE SOUNDTRACK: Paul Simon
In a pinch, I'd say Paul Simon's my favorite artist—either him or Neil Diamond, The Killers, Feist, Kanye West, Pearl Jam, Metric, Bad Brains, Jimmy Cliff, Willie Nelson, or Nas. I

messed up an interview with Neil Diamond once. I kept trying to ask him about the meaning of life, which makes it hard for someone to respond. With Paul Simon, I kept it simple—9/11, the future of Simon & Garfunkel, the meaning of life, and, of course, running songs. He gave me artists instead of individual records. What could I do? I said thanks.

Boozoo Chavis: "Some people don't know this zydeco musician from Louisiana, and that's a real shame."

Ali Farka Touré: "If you don't know Ali from Mali, that's something you want to check out. Ten years ago, he made records with Ry Cooder, who, by the way, is brilliant at understanding music from other cultures. He's done it many times brilliantly, including with a bunch of traditional Cuban artists. Their *Buena Vista Social Club* is another great album to own."

Celia Cruz: "The great Latin singer. All of her albums are great."

King Sunny Adé and Fela Kuti: "Great, great artists, who I've learned a lot from—neither of them are really new."

The Swan Silvertones: "I love the gospel quartets—the Silvertones and the Golden Gate Jubilee. Listen to the voices soar while you run."

The Delmore Brothers: "That's country music from the Grand Ole Opry. They influenced both Bob [Dylan] and me."

The Everly Brothers: "I also love the Delmore Brothers, the Louvin Brothers, and the Carter Family, but that's probably enough for now... How far are you trying to run?"

3

A FEW PROPER
WORDS ABOUT FORM

THE TRAINING: Halfway to Race Number One!

WEEK 6: Alternate running 6 minutes and walking 4 minutes for a total of 30 minutes, 3 times this week. (The proportions can change, obviously.)

WEEK 7: Three times, walk-run for 35 minutes, alternating 6 minutes of running with 4 minutes of walking for a total of 30 minutes and add 5 minutes of running at the end. When you're running more than walking, it's a beautiful thing.

THE SOUNDTRACK: Justin Bieber and Selena Gomez

THE FINISH LINE: A 5K race, now about 8 weeks away.

THE MAYOR of Toronto may or may not smoke crack. I never saw the video that supposedly shows him doing so. Together, we didn't smoke crack. What he does on his own time, I don't know. But he definitely weighs 330 pounds, and when we run together, he compliments me on my form. This is pretty weird, and not just because I'm bowlegged and land on my heels. The mayor hates the press, and although I don't cover city council—I cover sneakers—our going out for a jog together is a little like a pig taking a butcher to a Selena Gomez show. It just isn't done. However, here we are on the second-to-last day of the football season, and, although I've come looking for him at the high school by his house, the mayor receives me not as an enemy but as another poor bastard out here in the cold trying to work off a few pounds.

"Just have to make sure I don't get injured," mutters Mayor Ford, repeating every runner's gravest concern. The mayor has a running style that might best be described as an angry power-stride—head down, legs barely lifted, arms swinging side to side like a pissed-off Chubby Checker demonstrating the Twist. Ford's face is beet red and his breathing is labored; he looks like he'll need a defibrillator, not a Gatorade, when he's done. Oh, his stride isn't pretty—it's a plodding, determined stomp in the snow—but, as he says through heavy breathing, "I'm getting down."

"I gotta do it," he continues, and he's spot-on about that if he wants to join you in eight weeks for a 5K (3 miles).

This week and next, we're trying to reduce the proportions of how much you walk to how much you run. If you can run more efficiently, you won't have to work as hard. Which means limiting your jumping, twisting, skipping, heel-dragging, bending, zigzagging, clock-watching, and leaping. Go forward, not up, and only at red lights should you have both feet on the ground.

At first, your form's going to be whatever feels comfortable. When I watch the mayor trudge around the track in his sweatshirt, I can't tell him to land on the balls of his feet or to lean his torso slightly forward or to land under his hips and keep his elbows locked at right angles. The guy's doing everything he can to stay vertical, and he's losing a battle with his hefty frame to turn a walk into a jog. When I meet him, he's on lap eleven on his way to twenty. He has the hood up on his gray cotton sweatshirt, and his old sneakers are soaking. Work on your form? Yeah, right. I get it. After your boat capsizes is no time to demonstrate an elegant crawl.

"In the very beginning, you should work on endurance and find your natural rhythm," says Hal Higdon, who knows a thing or two about running. The author of thirty-six training books (and one racing novel), Higdon paid $3 to compete against 197 runners in the 1959 Boston Marathon, a race that now fields 26,000 people and costs $150 a bib ($200 if you're not a resident of the U.S.). Higdon is eighty years old and still running—he says he has perfect form—and he's recently begun a nice side business making oil paintings inspired by the races he's run.

"It got in my bones early and stuck," he says, adding that every runner's biomechanics are different and that some of the world's greatest runners also had some of the world's ugliest form. He rattles off the names of several top runners who exhibit "horrible, bad, ugly running," like Alberto Salazar, who won the Boston Marathon four times and now lives in Oregon, where he teaches form, among other things, to the world's best runners for Nike.

"Salazar was a mess, he was terrible, but he was also the world's best runner—nobody could beat him for years," Higdon says, proving the adage that whatever works, do that. According to Good Form Running, the official training website from New Balance (goodformrunning.com), proper technique has four elements: aligning your body with your feet under your hips, landing on the balls of your feet, aiming for a cadence of 180 steps per minute, and leaning slightly forward. Will you do all these things? Probably not, but it's absolutely something to shoot for. Same with concentrating on breathing deeply and rhythmically, and allowing your hands to hang loose. Unclench your fists, and let your arms swing. Keep your shoulders down, and away from your ears. Be relaxed, be conscious of your motions, and keep your back straight while bending your knees. And, oh yeah, have fun.

You're getting out there three times a week, pushing for thirty-five minutes: try different paces and body positions, and record your results. What feels best? That's what you should do. Basically, running is about concentration. This is why most elite runners don't listen to music. Focus on your movements and on getting from point A to point B in the smoothest possible fashion. Any herky-jerky actions will waste energy, and if you can keep your head and chin straight, your body should follow. Slightly tilt your neck back. "Once you get your head in place, work on your arms," says Higdon, adding that it's best if your arms swing in tandem with your landings: your right arm drops while your right foot lands, and if you don't swing your arms, your biceps will get tired from holding them up. Keep everything loose.

I understand it's an oxymoron to work out and be calm at the same time, but that's when the Zen comes in with long-distance running. When I'm running well, you could throw a football at me and I'd catch it. Of course, if I gave this advice to the mayor, he'd probably thwack me. When you're going as hard as you can, there's only one kind of form: get 'er done! But this will change. Sometimes, I can almost fall half-asleep while running and I feel like I can keep going forever. Form becomes innate; it's relaxing, it's rhythmic. It soothes. You just have to run a lot first. "Relaxation starts in the core of the body, from the stomach to the shoulder, which is why I tell new runners to take yoga," says Higdon. If you're breathing too hard, you're running too quickly, and, at least while starting, you should be able to maintain a conversation while you run.

At this point, you don't need to worry if you land on your heel or your midfoot. A piece in the *New York Times* estimated that more than 70 percent of runners land on our heels, which is fine. Lots has been made about the Kenyan midfoot style and barefoot running, which involves landing on the fleshy part of the foot behind the toes. Landing that way might help develop foot muscles and reduce the impact of landing, but then again, it might not.

If you want to get a sense of where Daniel Lieberman and the makers of Vibram FiveFingers think you should land, if you want to land on your midfoot, run backward. You'll come down on the balls of your feet. But there's no one right way to run, or at least, there's no one way that everyone should run. So for now, and quite possibly always, just do what comes naturally. And keep doing it. Keep up your schedule, and keep running. All you're doing now is playing with proportions, getting comfortable, and building routine and endurance. Keep decreasing how much of your thirty-five minutes you spend walking. Then do it again and again. I once asked Judd Apatow how to write a good screenplay and he told me, "Do it eight or nine or one hundred times." The same could be said about developing comfortable running form.

"WATCH LITTLE KIDS run around the playground, like little kids between the ages of eight and twelve. I tell my guys: Do that!" says Aaron Flamino, a high school cross-country track coach at Ellington High School in Ellington, Connecticut, just outside Hartford. "Little kids land flat-footed or with their midfoot, and the heel hits second. Since my guys are still learning their habits, we try to teach them to land with their foot under their hips." There's a difference between foot strike and foot placement and you'll be much more likely to connect on your midfoot if you land under your hips, Flamino told me. To hit the balls of your feet with your leg way extended, you'd need lots of hip flexion. Try to envision the running style of Groucho Marx. Flamino's a cool guy, plain-spoken, and a second-generation high school track coach, and he's used the family know-how to train his wife for the New York City Marathon. The coach is five-foot-eight, but he says that when he's running, he feels six feet tall.

"The most basic thing is to run like you're massive. You want your head to be high and your knees making nice vertical jags in the air," says Flamino, who teaches his kids proper running form by jogging up and down hills. "It's hard to run up a hill with bad form," he adds, telling me that when we run at an incline, our hamstrings, quads, and glutes do all the hard work, which is good, because they're our largest muscles. Flamino's constantly on his team to avoid "chicken wings," or elbows flailing out to the side. Good form is about aerodynamics—remember, you're listening to "Gangnam Style," not running that way—so you don't want to waste any motions. Since running is basically falling forward, a good stride means you're falling and catching yourself gracefully and everything's synchronized, like the components of a Pixar film. Draw power by swinging your arms forward, with your diaphragm open, eyes focused forward, and head straight, looking ahead.

"Kids on the playground—they aren't doing it for the exercise; they just love to run," says Flamino. "Attitude probably plays the biggest factor in form."

LOTS OF TIMES being a journalist takes me to places I would never otherwise go. Other members of the media travel to Syria or Afghanistan, and I may do that someday. But today,

I'm a guest of the Medcan Clinic in Toronto. My shirt is off, reflective markers are attached to my pelvis, and I'm hooked up to a computer to analyze my running form. I'm strapped into the same kind of contraption that animators used on Mike Myers to turn him into Shrek. If you want to run with geometric perfection—from the velocity of your peak tibial rotation (how quickly your lower leg twists inward) to the whip of your heel (how far your foot twists outward when it comes off the ground)—a gait analysis can measure every crook of your body and tell you how to improve. It's *Blade Runner* meets *Chariots of Fire*, and it's an ultramarathon away from a barefoot Kenyan or a kid playing in the park. "We're trying to transform an art form into a science," says Reed Ferber, director of the Running Injury Clinic at the University of Calgary and the inventor of the 3D gait-analysis system, which really could use a snappier name. "All of the research right now is related to injury treatment. This has everything to do with preventing injury in the first place."

The injury rate among runners is frightening. According to a 2002 study by Dr. Jack Taunton at the University of British Columbia, as many as 30 to 50 percent of runners get injured each year. This number hasn't changed since companies started compensating for pronation in their shoes. Ferber thinks most running injuries can be avoided.

How Most Running Injuries Can Be Avoided: A Survival Guide, by Reed Ferber

1. Stop buying into hype and marketing about fads, footwear, nutritional supplements, or running styles. Follow the research, but trust your own common sense.
2. Take enough time off between runs, and especially after long runs. Rest is sometimes more beneficial to your body than training, as it allows tissues to heal and recoup.

3. Run in a neutral cushioning shoe. Only 2 percent of all runners show signs of excessive pronation and need a motion-control shoe.

4. Listen to your body. Pain at the beginning of a run is OK. If the pain doesn't subside as the run continues, or if it gets worse or is painful when you stop your run, you are injured. Seek professional advice.

5. Realize and appreciate that running efficiently is based on strength, degree of flexibility, and anatomical structure. Once you change your running style, you become inefficient and put yourself at risk of injury. [Ed. note: Many would dispute this claim, however, and say that running's a skill like any other and that you can refine your technique, but it's Reed's list and, really, who knows?]

6. Strengthen your key stabilizer muscles (your core; see Chapter 21) to help maintain good form. A strong core keeps you stable; a weak core leads to muscle imbalances, which lead to injuries.

7. Develop a training plan and stick to it. Deviations from your plan are the proverbial "straw" that puts you over your injury threshold.

Your body compensates for muscular deficiencies, and how you twist and turn and carry your pelvis can indicate where you're going to be hurt. In a perfect world, you would reach your maximum pronation—the farthest inward curve in your foot when you land—at the halfway point of your stride. One foot's absorbing the bulk of the fall when your other foot's at the peak of its kick. Think about this stuff when you're running. Learn good habits now, when you're starting, before you go out on four-hour runs.

At Medcan, the markers on my pelvis report lots of information, none of it good. I jump too high and then lift my foot too quickly, before peak pronation, and my efficiency level is low. Since I spend too much time in the air, I compensate by rushing my motions on the ground, which means that I am not gaining maximum power when I take off with each foot rotation. Thus I lengthen my stride and have to work harder, and my form breaks down more quickly than it should. If you're running 42K (26 miles), the last thing you want to do is spend any more energy than you have to. I also rediscover that I'm bowlegged, and that when I try to run quickly I come dangerously close to knocking my knees. I get so much bad news I'm surprised that no one tells me that Greystone Books, my publisher, is bankrupt.

Not everyone's going to have a 3D gait analysis done, but the treadmill at your gym that's in front of the mirror is a good place to really take a look at how you run. When you push, you become fatigued. When you become fatigued, your form becomes more about survival than grace—like Mayor Ford on the race track—and when your form's crooked, you land strangely. "The runner who lasts is the one whose form deteriorates the least," says Dr. Andrew Miners, the sports injury specialist who leads me through Ferber's tests. "The right combination of biomechanics, functional movement, core strength, and stability is the trick for running a very long time."

I'd like to say Medcan was a revelation. I talk to Reed Ferber often, but in truth I just don't have the energy to change my form. I'm about to have my first child. I work for a newspaper. I've got a lot on my mind. I'm supposed to reduce my stride length because my steps per minute are 156, not the optimal 180, but I was never any good at math. Maybe you are.

Decide why you're running. Is it to maximize performance? Get some sun? Blow off steam? Your form is the gateway to a good finish, and by "good," I just mean finishing like this is something you might try again. You can't really run incorrectly—you can run stupidly, but you're only really running wrong if you smack into a bus. However, you can make it easier on yourself if you increase efficiency. Running, like nearly everything, is a lot more fun when you don't have to work as hard.

THE SOUNDTRACK, PART I: Justin Bieber
In person, Justin Bieber looks like a Justin Bieber doll. He wears a giant diamond-encrusted cross, earrings in both ears, and an oversized red Moschino T-shirt with baggy blue jeans. He's like this beautiful hip-hop baby, and you want to hug him. But the thing is, there's an Israeli security guard at the door and the kid's worth $112 million.

He just bought a $10-million home in the Hollywood Hills. Touch him, and his boys will lay you out. I got fifteen minutes with Bieber, and when he gave me a high five, he snapped his fingers afterward. That meant something to me. Did Bieber think I was cool?

He gave me two running songs:

"Dirty Diana," Michael Jackson: "Michael's definitely my biggest influence, and this song's good for crazy energy. I don't listen to someone else's music before I do a show—I just get out there and do it—but this song's really special. It's my pick for a running tune."

"You Make Me Wanna...," Usher: Bieber didn't say anything interesting about this Usher song, but he said something else that I like: "My tour sold out in one hour. My whole North American tour. I could've added more dates, but if I did, where's the demand? There's no demand, and people see that you go on tour all the time. If they miss you, they're like, That's cool, whatever. He'll be back. With me, you don't know if I'll be back. This might be your only chance."

WE FINISHED our interview, and then Bieber gave me my second high five of the morning. Afterward, we both added a snap.

THE SOUNDTRACK, PART II: Selena Gomez

I didn't interview Bieber with Gomez. In fact, when I interviewed the twenty-one-year-old Disney crossover star, who also had a bodyguard at the door and two publicists in the room, I was informed that there would be absolutely no Bieber questions. The two may or may not be an item. Since I wasn't allowed to ask her, and since I didn't know who she was when I met Bieber, I'll never know. Anyway, who cares about their love life? All I'm after is running songs. She gave us three: "'Run the World (Girls)' by Beyoncé, because we do run the world, that's a good one; Cheryl Cole, 'Fight for this Love,' and I'd say 'Toxic,' by Britney Spears."

"How about one of your songs?" I asked her.

"You should definitely run to 'Slow Down,'" she said.

I was going to tell her that's not the best message to send to a runner, but I couldn't. I ran out of time.

4

DETERMINATION, MOTIVATION, WOODY HARRELSON, AND DAVID SEDARIS

THE TRAINING: The No-Walk Test Drive

WEEK 8: Three times, walk-run for 35 minutes, alternating 2 minutes of walking with 8 minutes of running for a total of 30 minutes and add 5 minutes of running at the end.

WEEK 9: Run twice this week for 35 minutes, with a 1-minute walk at 10-minute intervals, and then run the entire final 5 minutes home.

WEEK 10: Now try 2 runs for 30 minutes without walking at all. It you can't do it, no problem. But it's better to experiment in practice than in a race.

THE SOUNDTRACK: Ghostface Killah

THE FINISH LINE: The 5K, now just about 6 weeks away.

WELCOME TO the guts of your 5K (3-mile) training program. By the end of Week 10, you may want to try running for a full thirty minutes without walking at all. You've been running for seven weeks now, completed about twenty runs, bought sneakers, and downloaded Justin Bieber's favorite Michael Jackson song. If your muscles feel sore, take a cold bath. It reduces soreness and mends tiny muscle tears. Also, if you don't want to spring for a sports drink, mix juice with water and add salt. You lose sodium when you sweat.

In Week 8, run three times, tweaking the walk-run ratio and running the entire final five minutes to your home. Then, in Week 9, run twice for thirty minutes, but run hard. Can you run for thirty minutes with only a one-minute walk break every ten minutes? Give it a shot and record the results. Finally, as you reach Week 10, run for thirty minutes without walking. If you can't do it, so what? Explore your boundaries. Besides, you should have a race goal. And you might as well pretend one of these practice runs is the real thing.

YOUR RACE is approaching, and it's imperative, if you've been slacking, not to double up on the workouts. That'll do more harm than good. You don't want an overuse injury and, even if you don't hurt yourself, there's no point showing up to the starting line exhausted. With race day in sight, be mindful. It's probably best to skip ribfest and maybe ease off on the daiquiries for the next few nights. Remember: races are timed. You will arrive at a starting line with lots of other runners. When the run's over, people will ask you how you did. So everything between now and race day is important. Give yourself a chance to succeed.

THE MOST famous coach in college distance running is much more impressed with you—the casual first-time runner—than he thinks you should be with him or his athletes. Mark Wetmore of the University of Colorado Buffaloes is the only NCAA Division 1 track coach to win all four cross-country titles—team victories and individual golds for both men and women—in the history of the sport. Since 2000, his teams have won five championships, and, in his spare time, he's privately coached another fifty-one athletes to gold. An eccentric—he's as influenced by Ken Kesey as he is by Steve Prefontaine—the guy's taken eight Colorado Buffaloes to the Olympics and boasts a record so impressive that his methods were featured in a book called *Running with the Buffaloes*, which detailed the coach and his team. Wetmore, known for marching his troops up the 425-meter (1,400-foot) incline of Flagstaff Mountain, is himself a former distance champion. Still, he's not one to blow his own shoes. Not when asked about the challenges faced by people who are just six weeks away from their first 5K.

"So many of those weekend warriors who train before work or, particularly in my opinion, who come home from a long day of work and change and go out the door, I admire their motivation. They're more motivated than many collegiate athletes who have everything placed on the table in front of them," says Wetmore, now in his thirty-third year of professional distance coaching. "I can't think of anything more difficult than to leave a long day of work and go home, and down one hallway is the refrigerator and down the other hall are your running shoes. I don't know how you do it, actually."

So how do you do it? How do you stay motivated and stick to a plan when there's no prize for what you accomplish, and whether you run or not won't affect the relationship between Selena and Justin?

Eleven ways to stay motivated with running:

1. Sign up for a race.
2. Reverse your training route.
3. Buy new sneakers.
4. Find a running group.

5. Incorporate speed drills into your workout so that you will run faster. Which is to say: instead of running for thirty minutes, run for ten, but go as fast as you can.
6. Update the playlist on your iPod.
7. For instance, add "Survivor" by Destiny's Child. Alanis Morissette, who ran the New York City Marathon in 2009, told me that when she hit Mile 20, she played that song twenty times in a row.
8. Record all your workouts.
9. Look at yourself naked in front of the mirror. Perhaps there's something you'd like to change?
10. Challenge somebody, anybody, to a race.
11. Reward yourself amply when you're through.

To some degree, running has to have an intrinsic value. Hopefully, running makes you feel good. You've obviously set out on this path to accomplish something, and whether it's to cross the marathon off your bucket list, lose some weight, or if not give up, at least reduce, the late nights at the pub, you're now well on your way toward your race. And that's why events are important. You'll be less inclined to quit if you have a specific goal in mind, and much less inclined to quit if you've shelled out for sneakers and told all your friends that you're running 5K.

"There's no use getting all hot and bothered about some exciting goal that's totally impossible, but if you want to do this, go out the door slowly and in the back of your mind, keep thinking about that goal," says Wetmore. "The important thing is that you're able to do it, and do it again and again."

LEARNING HOW to run, and sticking with the training, has parallels in the everyday world. It's the difference between love at first sight and being married with kids. You have to work beyond the initial thrill. When David Sedaris wanted to become a writer, he kept a strict schedule, rewarded himself amply, and stuck to it. This is never easy to do. But Sedaris, echoing Wetmore, says it's much harder for the amateur, the person first starting out, than it is for someone who knows the drill: "I've always been pretty good about doing the exact same thing at the exact same time, but it's hard when it's a hopeless enterprise. It's easy for me now to get up tomorrow morning and write because I have an audience—I know another book will come out—but when I started, not only did I have no outlet, but I sucked and I knew how bad I was," Sedaris says. He adds: "It's hard at the beginning to keep faith."

Faith, of course, is at the root of any worthwhile endeavor—from starting a band to bringing a new life into the world. It takes faith to start running and go after the marathon. And the belief you need is belief in yourself. It helps, though, if you pad your journey with rewards along the way. For me, there's no better taste than my cold Gatorade fruit punch out of a tin thermos in the summer after I've completed my 20K morning run.

Treats come in various shapes and sizes—some healthy, some not so much. Harley Pasternak, who trains Megan Fox, Kanye West, and Kim Kardashian, isn't a fan of running. He thinks runners are prone to walk around the block and then reward themselves with a banana split. Keep perspective. But if you run a lot, you can eat a lot too. Plus, your appreciation of things we often take for granted is enhanced after a run: a grapefruit seems sweeter, a glass of water more refreshing, even your chair feels more comfortable.

Make sure you take the time to acknowledge your achievements; that's one reason it's important to write everything down. If you chart your progress, you're more likely to keep progressing. And if you can see something's working—and you document that, yes, now I run more than I walk—you're more likely to stick with it. It's a big deal to switch the ratio between walking and running. Just like it's a big deal to run outside and a big deal to enter a race. There will be frustrating moments and setbacks. The point is: notice the good stuff. Every time you run just a little bit farther or a little bit faster, appreciate what you're doing: you're getting closer to your goal.

YOU'RE NOW getting comfortable with running for around thirty-five minutes, which is about how long the average woman takes to run 5K. That average 5K female finisher is a shade over thirty-three years old and may or may not have run the distance before. (Surely the average of first-timers only would be longer than thirty-five minutes.) Meanwhile, the average guy finishes in twenty-seven minutes and is forty-two years old.

When you're running, get a sense of what thirty-five minutes feels like. And use mapmyrun.com, a pedometer, Google maps, or the odometer in your car to measure how far you're actually going. It's possible you're already doing 5K.

DIFFERENT PEOPLE run for different reasons. Wesley Korir, winner of the 2012 Boston Marathon, said, "If you're not running for something, then you're just chasing the wind." Find your purpose. Mary Keitany is a Kenyan athlete who was one of the fastest female runners in the world. Until she had her baby. Then she became one of the fastest women of all time.

"To be a professional runner who can make money in running—it can change your life and change the life of your family too," Keitany tells me from her home in Kenya, where she's married to the competitive marathon racer Charles

Koech. "Kenya is a poor country, and the people use running to buy your house and have money in your pocket. Since I became a mother, I have more responsibility. I need to run well to give a good future for my son." In 2011, Keitany ran the half-marathon in the United Arab Emirates in 1:05:50 and set a world record. She won the London Marathon in 2011 and 2012, picking up $55,000 each time. She runs not only for her life but for her son's life as well.

You will never run as fast as Mary Keitany. Among other things, you don't train as hard, because you don't have to. After Keitany runs, she eats something healthful and then takes a nap. When she wakes up, she has tea and goes out for another run. After that, she calls it a day. You probably can't make that kind of commitment. But you still need to find a recipe that works because it can be damn hard getting off the couch.

"I'm a lazy son of a bitch, I can't lie," says Woody Harrelson, eyes red, smile mischievous, when I meet him in a tiny community theater in Toronto where he's launching *Bullet for Adolf*, an autobiographical play. "If I can put something off to the last minute—or let's be honest here, a good two or three decades—I will." I know the feeling. Most of us are lazy. And if we aren't lazy, we're pooped. We work too much and we're busy. I'm tired. God knows how Julie feels working as a producer, not sleeping, and carrying around a little Julie for the past seven months. It's kind of like what Colorado coach Mark Wetmore said: If you've got a job and a family, who has the time—let alone the inclination—to put something more, something grueling, and something with benefits you might not see right away, on your plate? Running gives me energy, but, when I'm exhausted, that can be difficult to believe.

Harrelson's been nominated for two Oscars, and of course he earned his stripes on *Cheers*, but the guy I meet in the local theater is just another schlub who's been putting something off for the past twenty-eight years. "The question isn't how long have I been working on this play, it's how long have I not been," he says, glassy eyed, sheepishly looking at the ground. "Sometimes it's easier to find a reason not to do something than to actually get something done."

So how did he get from the page to the stage, in essence from not running at all to completing his first marathon? The same way you're going to get to 5K. Harrelson dedicated himself to a routine and committed—full stop—to a detailed plan. And by assigning himself achievable goals throughout the process—from writing a few pages to producing a first draft to scheduling a reading with actors to raising the curtain—Harrelson arrived at his finish line. "I just couldn't have lived with myself if I'd put it off any longer," says Harrelson, himself a runner battling a bum knee. (He's a fan of *Born to Run* and a devotee of the Vibram FiveFingers barefoot shoes.) "I said, 'This is it. I'm not stopping. I'm going to do it this time'—and I did."

The way I keep myself running is by finding new finish lines and keeping a standing appointment with Ben every Tuesday and Thursday, no matter what the weather might be. Races are like tests, which get students to keep up with their homework. If you pay money to compete in a thing, you really shouldn't back out. And since you're not backing out, you really should take a good crack at whatever it is you choose to do. The races I run justify the hours I spend on my training, and even though the outcome doesn't matter, I'm motivated by having a certain time that I'm trying to beat. For me, that challenge helps keep running from getting monotonous. Jogging is mindlessly going around and around in circles. Running is doing something purposeful, with a plan. Marathoners often talk about being focused when they run. They're not just asleep out there as they're kicking; they're working, pushing themselves, paying attention to their body, their breathing, their form. Do that, and before you know it, you might start enjoying these weekly runs. Push forward, and you'll lose so much weight you'll need a smaller-sized shoe. Keep running, and one day you'll wake up and it's happened—you've become Forrest Gump.

Harrelson picks up his story: "I was freaking out, man. There was a scene at the end of the first act that was driving me bananas. It wasn't right, and I was losing my mind," he says, adding that he blocked and reblocked the scene, changed the script, and asked for input from his actors. It was neither quick nor easy, but eventually, he accomplished his goal. "I feel pretty satisfied, man. I mean, you never know what people will say, but we had a job to do and I think we did it real well," he says. "This was hanging around my neck for a long while, and while it wasn't easy, what can I tell you? We saw the old son of a bitch through."

Motivation is what gets you out of the house. Determination is what takes you down a pant size. Together, these two characteristics made David Sedaris a great writer. And they got Woody Harrelson off-Broadway. And they'll see you through your training and across your finish line too.

THE SOUNDTRACK: Ghostface Killah
"On the way out, they hit me up real quick; they got me out of the car and frisked me—they didn't handcuff me, though," says Ghostface Killah from the Wu-Tang Clan, as my daughter bounces up and down on my lap, yelling at the top of her lungs. I'm recording all this so it's kosher, but it seems incredible that a) I finally have Ghost on the phone after twenty-eight attempts and b) that, when I do, I'm watching my daughter

who's screaming as he tells me about his experience with the Canadian cops.

Ghost, who was going by the name Ironman Tony Starks while Robert Downey Jr. was still waking up at his neighbor's house in Malibu, has never run a marathon, but his description of what it feels like to be onstage matches how you should think of yourself when you race.

"I'm thinking: I'm king. This is my house—I own this shit and whatever I say goes," he says. "People try and do what I do, but that's all they can do, imitate. It's very rare—very rare—to find someone who knows how to do what I do, and when it comes to an actual performance? People get kind of nervous trying to stand next to me." He isn't happy to be recommending running songs—next question, he says more than once—but I walk around Toronto in a Ghostface T-shirt. I had to get his running songs in the book.

"Louder than a Bomb," Public Enemy: "Listen to that break beat, the horn, the siren. People are all on 'Don't Believe the Hype,' but this joint, with the repeats right there and the Flavor chorus? I don't really jog, I walk on the treadmills and ride the bike in the gym, but this could be some theme music right there: 'Louder than a Bomb.'"

"Daytona 500," Ghostface Killah: "You need fast tracks with those kinds of angry tear-your-head-off type beats. We have so many of those records [raps part of his verse from "Daytona 500"]: *In the Philippines, pick herbal beans, bubblin' strings/ Body chemical 'Cream,' we burn kerosene.* That's racing music right there, kid."

"Run," Ghostface Killah: "That's the anthem. You can run to that joint all day."

5

24 HOURS BEFORE
THE START LINE

THE TRAINING: Mixed Taper

WEEK 11: Run 3 times for 30 minutes with a 90-second walk (if needed) in the middle. Sunday, 7 days before race day, should be your last hard run.

WEEK 12: Taper. If the race is Sunday, don't run past Thursday, though walk, bike, or do yoga to keep active (you don't want tired muscles but you don't want rested muscles either). Two 20-minute jogs will keep you sharp, but not exhausted. After 3 months, one more day of training more won't make you faster but it can tire out your legs.

THE SOUNDTRACK: Broken Social Scene

THE FINISH LINE: The 5K, now just about 3 weeks away!

RATHER THAN my telling you about what to do in your holy last hours before the starting line, I'm going to let Deena Kastor share her tips. No big deal, she's just the fastest American female marathon runner of all time, and, oh yeah, the all-time fastest American woman in the half-marathon, too.

How I Spend My Last Waking Moments Before Racing: A Love Story, by Deena Kastor

6:00 a.m.: Wake up, and drink a big glass of water.

6:15: Have a cup of coffee, a couple of pieces of toast, and watch the Weather Channel. I make sure I don't have a chill, because it uses up glycogen (see Chapter 7).

7:00: Go for a shake-out run of four or five miles. I don't wear a watch or set a pace, I just go with whatever feels good.

7:30: Run a portion of the route. Come race day, when I hit that portion, it gives me exhilaration. I like that familiarity.

9:30: Get a light stretch and massage. If you don't have the luxury, like me, of a husband who will do it for you, sit on the ground and stretch whatever feels tight.*

11:15: Eat an early lunch. Since the evening meal is bland, for lunch I'll have a turkey sandwich with vegetables or a pizza with vegetables, something with a little excitement.

12:30 p.m.: Watch television or get on the computer, but don't do anything business-related. I don't want to focus on anything other than the race. I scan websites for decorating ideas. And I try not to be on my feet too much.

1:00 to 3:00: Ahhh, nap.

3:00: Get outside, and get some fresh air. I might walk the dog or sit in the shade by the pool or in the park. It's hard to say how much time goes by because I do everything at a leisurely pace. The day's going to feel eternal. [Ed. note: Deena Kastor is what's known as an elite, a runner who races professionally. For us non-elites, the day's spent picking up our race bib, laying out our clothing, packing a postrace bag, studying the course map, figuring out where the water stations—and our cheerleaders—will be, and planning our route to the start line. Note: the day doesn't feel eternal.]

5:00: Eat a long meal. Pesto pasta and a little salmon is my ideal, with a nice glass of red wine. It helps me sleep better and relax.

7:30: Go to bed.

8:00: Fall asleep. (I have no problem lying down with the sun still in the sky. Maybe that's just an attribute of any tired mother.)

4:00 a.m.: Get up four hours before race time. Drink a large glass of water.

4:25: Do a couple of skips to wake up, get dressed, and head down for breakfast in running shoes.

4:40: Eat an early breakfast. I like espresso, a toasted bagel with butter, and scrambled eggs. (If I'm traveling and can't get scrambled eggs, I'll make hardboiled eggs the day before and put them in a resealable plastic bag set over ice.) I like an early breakfast so I have time to digest.

5:15 to 6:15: Sit around and stay off my legs. I pin my number to my shirt and make sure the timing chip is on my shoe correctly while I watch the Weather Channel. I'm obsessed with dressing warmly enough.

7:00: On the bus to the race, I surround myself with the people I'm most comfortable with. I bring a trash bag because if it's wet I don't want to sit on the ground.

7:15: Talk to people. I love running because of the community.

7:29: On the starting line, I tune into the fluttering in my stomach and try to breathe into the queasiness. I feel like I'm going to throw up. My hands are shaking, but I'm not nervous. Being nervous has negative connotations. I'm excited. It's energy, and being excited is positive.

7:30: Run!

* If your hips feel tight, try sitting down on the floor, feet together, and elbows gently applying pressure down on your thighs.

If your quadriceps feel tight, try standing on one foot, bending your knee, and raising the foot behind you.

If your hamstrings feel tight, try sitting on the floor with your legs out straight, and your arms reaching forward toward your toes.

If your back feels tight, try sitting with your legs shoulder-width apart. Extend your arms, cross your left bicep over your right, and bend your elbows. Your right forearm should catch your left elbow. Now twist to your right side and hold the pose for twenty seconds. Repeat on the other side.

TWO WEEKS from race day, hit your three runs with purpose. Take two runs for thirty minutes and try to envision the race. Scare yourself. How fast can you go and sustain that speed for 5K (3 miles)? In Week 12, there's no need to do much more than twenty minutes, and definitely don't run more than that when you're forty-eight hours from your race. Up until Sunday, a week from race day, is the time to test yourself. Then, with the countdown less than one week away, taper. Run twice, but exercise caution and listen to your body. If you're exhausted, go for ten minutes. If you feel good, go twice for twenty minutes and run hard for a minute at five-minute intervals. This will keep your muscles sharp and engaged. But only you know your condition. And it's better, a week from race day, to be cautious than brave.

Most races take place on a Sunday, so don't run past Thursday during your taper week, but stay active: take a bike ride, walk, use the stairs, try yoga, go for a swim. You don't want to do anything here that you don't usually do, or kill a pint of Häagen-Dazs, or drop acid at a Carrie Underwood show. The important thing is to feel fit, and the mind game is key. The saying goes that you can't do anything on race day that you haven't done in practice. This doesn't exactly hold for 5K, because when you're starting to run the tendency is to be over-cautious. Also, there's race-day magic—like how a mother can knock out a grizzly if it threatens her kid—but don't plan on this special juju. You might find a Picasso at a yard sale, but c'mon, it's out there but best forgotten. And this is why racing is awesome: you don't know what you can do until tested.

For now, though, chilling is the best prerace medicine. Deena Kastor doesn't even look at her office computer the day before a big race. It makes no sense to show up exhausted to the starting line. Instead, figure out how far your thirty-five-minute runs have taken you. And once you figure out how far you've been running, figure out how long it takes. From there, you can determine your average pace. I write these split times on my hand. (And, unfortunately, tend to ignore them during the race. Pacing, even when not wearing sneakers, is hard.)

The more information you have about what to expect, the more relaxed you'll be. And you'll likely go faster on race day than you have in practice, both because you'll be able to run continuously without having to stop for red lights and because people cheering you on gives you an enormous endorphin boost. Instead of just having to squeeze a jog in, on race day, the jog is the thing. Listen to Carey Pinkowski: "The fun part of the event is the unpredictability. Surprise yourself, because the beauty of a race is—you never know."

"Familiarize yourself with the basics. How are you getting to the race? Where are you parking? Where, after the race, are you meeting your friends?" says Pinkowski, race director of the Chicago Marathon, which attracts around 40,000 competitors, brings in something like $220 million to the local economy, produces 1,310 jobs, and, in 2011, raised $13 million for charity. "Racing is hard, so experienced runners make everything else easy. Pick out your clothing the night before; don't wear anything you haven't worn before; and, whatever you do, don't eat anything different. I always advise racers to turn a practice run into a dry run of the race, then just repeat what works on race day."

If you're entered in a popular race, it's going to be crowded when you arrive, cacophonous. And lots of people are going to be ducking into the bushes to pee. Race bibs are generally colored, and the color on your bib corresponds to the estimated finishing time you filled out on the race entry form. The race organizers want the fastest runners up front so slower runners won't be crushed in a stampede. You're placed in corrals. If you estimated your time correctly, there shouldn't be tons of people passing you. Look for the corral that corresponds to your bib color, and plan to get there about twenty-five minutes before start time. Do you get cold easily? Deena Kastor brings a garbage bag; I don't—but it's your call. When you're in the corral, just breathe easy. By now your iPod's charged, and you're ready. Think of the nerves as positive vibes.

"The first time you do a race, it's not about how fast you can run but what you can learn," says Roger Moss, coach of

Toronto's Longboat Roadrunners, one of Canada's oldest and largest running clubs. This is true always, but especially true at your first 5K. Remove the pressure. You've never done this before. You're not an expert. It's fine to walk, to stop, to ask for help. The goal isn't to run once and despise the experience. The race is the culmination of a challenging three months. Of course, the running itself won't be easy. But what is? Remember, this is just a first stop on a long-ass journey. You'll do this again, so relax.

After all, as Kathrine Switzer says, "This is a celebration, nothing to be nervous about." She knows about racing jitters. In 1967, when she became the first woman to register for and complete the Boston Marathon, a psychotic race official tried wrestling her to the ground. "You can be bitter or you can be inspired, but I choose to feel inspired," she tells me. "It's hard to run when you're mad." You have your health. You have the time to run and the time, afterward, to recover. You're lucky, some might even say blessed. So if you can tap into those emotions, feeling happy, feeling appreciative, feeling alive, you might find something more than a good workout.

It's not just another day at Costco and it's not getting slowly squeezed out at work. Pay tribute to your training and your accomplishments. You've worked hard. If there's water being handed out by volunteers, grab a cup. If a stranger applauds you, give 'em five.

THE SOUNDTRACK: Broken Social Scene
I didn't love Toronto when I first moved here. I may have been answering the phones at *GQ*, but at least I had my own apartment. When I arrived in Canada, I found myself unemployed and living in Julie's parents' house. Eventually, as happens, I went about solving my relocation problems, and a big part

of that was making some friends, finding some employment, and getting involved with the city's music world. In Toronto, this is Broken Social Scene.

Kevin Drew and Brendan Canning, the band's leaders, aren't exactly my friends. I don't call them up to babysit Esme, but it's been eight years I've known them now and seen them out, been to their shows, written about their records, and I've come to see our relationship as a symbol of the life Julie and I have made in Toronto. And it's good. Their music is epic, guitar-driven, romantic, and dense. I was pleased when they recommended some tunes.

First, Kevin Drew:

"Bound to Be That Way," Do Make Say Think: "I'm a huge Do Make Say Think fan, and I can tell you that your life will be better if you listen to this band. When you start your run, put on *You, You're a History in Rust*. The first song is 'Bound to Be That Way,' and there's a rise and fall and rise again, and that's what running is about. It's a soundtrack. The first song is a warm-up, but then the album progresses: there's melodies, crescendos, and everything's raw. This record could be the sound of your body."

"Rock 'n' Roll Damnation," AC/DC: "I also recommend 'Rock 'n' Roll Damnation' by AC/DC, off *Powerage*, just for the shaker alone, although they have the greatest rhythm section of all time. Outstanding. I got into DC when I was four and never looked back."

Now, Brendan Canning, who also DJs and, though when he runs he doesn't listen to music, designed a quick little mix:

Start: Curtis Mayfield, "Future Shock": "The tempo's not too fast, but it's got enough drive to get ya moving—shocking the body."

Get Pumping: Metallica, "Fight Fire with Fire": "Gettin' mad. Fake out acoustic intro and then POW!"

Get Tired: Erik Satie, "Gymnopédie No. 1": "Zen out. Don't put too much pressure on yourself. Enjoy the burn."

Rally: Subway, "Persuasion": "Great continuation from Satie… still Zen, but now getting that third wind… the beat kicks in and you're off!"

Finish Line: Public Enemy, "Burn Hollywood Burn": "Something to get you real mad. Even if you like Hollywood flicks, by the time Big Daddy Kane drops his line: *Aunt Jemima is the perfect term/Even if now she got a perm*, you have reached deep into the endorphin pockets."

6

RACE ONE,
RUNNING ANGRY:
OTTAWA

WHEN I arrive at the starting line for the Ottawa Race Weekend 10K, the first race in my year-long bid to run Boston, there's a herd of teenagers in front of me, in the wrong corral, in the wrong clothing, yelling and blocking my path. I mill about, hungover, stewing in my own negative juices, and strike up a conversation with a guy in knee-high compression socks. I have my kilometer split times written on my hand, as always, and I'm hoping to come in under thirty-seven minutes, which would break all my previous personal records at this distance. Really, my time goals are geared only for the marathon, because I need to run 3:10 in October to qualify for Boston in April, so I use these shorter distances as speed tune-ups.

How long do you think it'll take you to finish 5K (3 miles)? I don't know. I always set my goals too high. My previous best in 10K (6 miles) is 37:39, even though it was on a downhill course in Toronto, but I feel like breaking myself out here today. I like going nuts. What's the absolute fastest I can run? The guy in the socks says thirty-seven is too fast for him. He's been too busy to train properly, and he'll be happy if he comes in under thirty-nine. "See you at the finish line," I tell him, and when the gun goes off, I dash by the kids. I like making races into wars.

I run my first kilometer in something like 3:30, and I'm flying, hitting the ground like it said something bad about my wife, but then a strange thing happens—it's like every kilometer between two and nine is mislabeled. Surely these vast distances are more than 1K long. I can hold on for a while, but I never establish a groove. I speed up, I slow down, and this wastes energy. People I passed at the start trot by me as we push beyond 6K (3 miles).

While I'm in Ottawa for the race, Julie, pregnant, is back home in Toronto with our expansive, expensive to-do list, including a change table that needs assembling. I didn't leave under the best conditions. We had invited people over for dinner last night, but I was late arriving home. I'd been teaching a run class, and the speaker I'd invited went on and on about the right way to wear a running bra. On the way home I forgot the dessert, and so when Julie had to run out for pastries, I ran headlong into the rum.

A day later, at 7K (4 miles), I can now feel the warm Bacardi sweat seeping through my pores. I know the race is almost over. I feel like a kid sitting in the dentist's chair: I just want it to be through. At worst, I can run four-minute kilometers (about six-and-a-half minutes per mile) and so I just need to keep on for another twelve minutes, and I'm like Rain Man, running the numbers in my head. But it feels like there's an anchor attached to my shoes. Guilt? I'm wearing good sneakers, the Brooks Ghosts recommended by Samantha Danbert, but I don't feel free and the sun doesn't give me power and I feel like a tired, creaky old bag of bones. The shoes seem to be loaded with concrete.

Here comes that jackass in the socks. "You're almost there, keep fighting!" he cheers. I grit my teeth, pick my head up, and give chase. Run like an eight-year-old girl playing tag? Be appreciative? Run with joy? Yeah right, asshole. I've got Bacardi streaming down my face.

I went out too quick, too soon, and I can't catch the sock man. Between 8 and 9K (4 and 5.5 miles), I run a bit faster and I give everything I have to that sacred last kilometer and cross the finish line at 38:55, disappointed—even though finishing under forty minutes is fast and I haven't been training and, as usual, don't follow my own advice. There's a lot of stuff I know about racing and running, and even more that I don't actually listen to but know I should.

You shouldn't run like me. You should run better. Good luck.

TWO

BUILDING ENDURANCE

REACHING 10K

"You can handle anything for
a short period of time."

LAURA SAMARAS, prenatal course instructor,
St. Joseph's Hospital, Toronto

WHAT WE TALK ABOUT WHEN WE TALK ABOUT SPAGHETTI

THE TRAINING: Thwarting the After-Race Blahs

WEEK 14: Run twice this week, 25 minutes each time, without any walking (though walk, of course, if you have to— perhaps 1 minute of walking for every 5 minutes you jog).

WEEK 15: Re-establish consistency by making this a 3-run week. Run twice for 25 minutes and once for 35 minutes. As ever, the most important thing is not to skip a run.

THE SOUNDTRACK: Kendrick Lamar

THE FINISH LINE: The 10K, now just about 13 weeks away.

TO RUN WELL, you have to fuel your body. As you begin to prepare for your 10K (6-mile) race, eating healthfully becomes even more critical. Carbohydrates, especially those with a low glycemic index, or GI, are particularly important. The GI measures how quickly carbohydrates are converted into blood glucose, the sugar that circulates in your bloodstream and is the body's main source of energy. Glucose, called glycogen when it enters the muscles, is what we burn first while we exercise. While training, you want to eat foods that combine complex carbohydrates and a low GI number—which are usually one and the same—because you want food that will sustain you rather than turning instantly to sugar. These foods tend to be boring and brown, and healthy and easy to digest, things like lentils and beans. Bran's also a good source of low-GI carbohydrates. Think about it: when we're running long distances, we don't want a sugar high. Better are foods with starch, which can be stored in the liver and muscles and dispersed through the body over time. A package of Junior Mints—which, like watermelon and white bread, are on the upper end of the GI scale—will turn into glucose and fuel our cells, but their sugar's consumed very quickly. The best stuff, like multigrain pastas, which contain whole wheat but also every bit of the grain kernel, including the fibers that contain bran, dispense energy over time. Foods like brown bread, unsweetened cold cereals, bagels, pita bread, sweet potatoes, and multigrain rice act almost like time-released energy capsules. This stuff will fill your glycogen reserves and keep you from hitting the Wall. What else should you eat instead of candy corn, Wonder Bread, and Popeyes? Apples, plums, and pears.

The thing about diet is the thing about training is the thing about race strategy: have a plan and keep yourself under control. My tendency is to go without and then gorge when I determine it's time to go with. It's binge and purge, or lots of steps forward and then one giant step back. You probably already know your worst instincts. Perhaps you intend to use running to keep them at bay?

NICOLE YUEN is a dietician just a few months away from her second half-marathon, and her first in San Francisco. Even when she's not running, she wears a Nike chip on her shoes. She and I are looking at the food in a 7-Eleven convenience store, and she does not recommend the pink Sno Balls. "I honestly can't think of any reason to eat a Twizzler," says Yuen, who walks me very slowly through the aisles, assessing the wares. She takes a moment to rethink her initial prognosis. "Maybe if you're at a party and want to indulge, but there's no nutritional benefit. And I just don't see the point of white bread." Yuen became interested in healthy eating after her father suffered a heart attack. Today, thanks to her, her old man no longer eats fatty cuts of meat from his favorite restaurants.

"Nutrition's about finding that moment when you're reaching for a donut in the morning and pulling your hand back and reaching for the cereal instead," says Jennifer Nelson, director of clinical dietetics at the Mayo Clinic in Minnesota and one of the principal authors of *The Mayo Clinic Diet*, which debuted at number one on the *New York Times* bestseller list when it was released in 2010. "Healthy eating's about finding those momentary motivations so when you're going to dig into the freezer and grab the ice cream, instead you open the fridge and grab a fruit. The more you get into the rhythm, the easier it gets." Eating cleanly is habit-forming. Buy groceries and pack your lunch. Buy groceries that are good for you. It's about small, incremental choices toward a clear, well-defined goal. You don't have to become a raw food devotee, but just chill out on the Monte Cristo sandwiches and prepared tomato sauce.

Brian Wansink, director of Cornell's food and brand lab and the author of *Mindless Eating*, says being aware of what we're consuming is the first step toward impulse control. "You can't say you're a victim of marketing. We all know what a double bacon cheeseburger does, and we're our own worst enemies," says Wansink, a frontline fighter trying to change the way Americans eat. In 2009, he spruced up the fruit displays in cafeterias across 1,300 American schools. He tells me he wants to get his healthy-eating program into 3,000 elementary schools by 2015. "The problem we have is our own bad habits," he says. "We try rewarding ourselves with food: I had a HUGE day, so I'm not having a piece of wheat toast for dinner. But that doesn't really make sense. Why would you reward yourself with a punishment?"

Nicole Yuen and I walk into the grocery store, and I ask her to fill my cart. She brings back oatmeal, bananas, whole-grain bread and pasta, skinless chicken breast, salad greens, natural peanut butter, low-fat Greek yogurt, nuts, fish, brown rice, and lentils. Most of the stuff she chooses is common sense. You know scarfing five Italian sausages is different from eating olive oil on wheat toast. The question is: How much effort do you want to put in to making those choices? Do you want your rewards now, or later?

Sometimes, when I want to bury my worst impulses, I pretend Nas is watching. It turns out that this is a good method for controlling your diet. Brian Wansink recently completed a study of six-year-olds in which he had them look through a pack of trading cards and pick out their favorite superhero. Afterward, he asked the kids to choose between carrot sticks and french fries. More than 50 percent chose carrots when also asked what their superhero would eat. "The same thing works with adults who are training for a half-marathon," says Wansink, a father of three and former executive director of the USDA's Center for Nutrition Policy and Promotion. "Imagine yourself crossing the finish line before you sit down at the table or else think about Ryan Hall or a Kenyan runner you admire, then ask yourself: Would this person have another scoop of ice cream?"

Babe Ruth ate hot dogs before baseball games, Frank Shorter had pizza the day before he won the 1972 Olympic gold medal and launched the first running boom, and you can have tacos and finish 10K. But nutrition plays a role not only in how you finish a race, but also in how you feel afterward. "If you pay attention to your nutrition before and during the race, it will make a big difference in not only whether you complete that marathon, but what your time will be and how destroyed you'll be at the end," says Dr. Raylene Reimer, a professor in the Department of Biochemistry and Molecular Biology at the University of Calgary, and a member of the Canadian Society of Clinical Nutrition. "It's never made sense to me that people will spend so much time picking out their race clothes, follow a great schedule for their training, then totally ignore what they use for their fuel."

According to Dr. Reimer, the Wall—that moment in a long-distance race when you feel like each sneaker's attached to your coffin—is a result of poor nutrition. The Wall occurs when the glycogen in your liver and your muscles gets depleted. "Eating foods high in carbohydrates the week before a race is important," she says, adding that energy gels and sports drinks during a long run help to boost glycogen. "During exercise, the digestive system isn't getting all the blood flow—the blood goes to the muscles—and so stocking up on complex carbohydrates gives you good glucose to help fight fatigue."

In addition to proper fueling, there's another dietary concern: finding yourself thirty minutes into a run being plagued by an irresistible urge to move your bowels. This situation is natural and afflicts even the most experienced runners. In Toronto, when Reid Coolsaet qualified for the Olympics, he had to stop during the race to take a shit. (He had just started drinking beet juice, for the oxygen, but learned about the side effects too late.) Coolsaet, however, wasn't concerned. This is such a normal occurrence that during the most important race of his life, he'd stuffed toilet paper into his shorts. (Something I'm sure Paula Radcliffe wished she had done during her televised pit stop by the side of the road at the 2005 London Marathon. Google it, or don't.)

Everyone's digestive system is different. For me, dairy opens the floodgates like a levee in New Orleans. On mornings when I run, I eat English muffins with peanut butter and a banana, along with a cup of coffee and a glass of orange juice. (I've also ruined a brand-new pair of bright yellow shoes, and I'm embarrassed to say what's happened to more than one pair of socks.) "Running gets the intestines moving; that peristaltic rhythmic contraction kicks in, and you feel the call of nature," says Reimer, imploring runners to avoid bran muffins, beans, or anything else that's high in fiber on race day. "Anything that can cause the intestines to move more frequently—apricots, prunes—those are the kinds of foods to avoid." Reimer says you don't have to avoid your morning coffee, though; it's not a strong diuretic unless you consume five to seven cups, and new research shows caffeine—from coffee, chocolate, or sport drinks and gels—can actually give runners a competitive edge.

Avoiding the bad stuff and selecting the good stuff will make you a better runner, but be kind to yourself. No one's saying that to run the half-marathon you need to commit to a diet of exclusively whole wheat and lentils. "I married a guy who loves fast food, but the restaurants always want to enlarge your portion sizes and encourage you to keep adding to your order. It's like, OK, enough!" says Paula Cantu, the director of Nutrition Services at Arlington Memorial Hospital and a former marathon runner. Cantu, who supervised a weight-loss program for overweight soldiers in Fort Sill, Oklahoma, says she's OK with letting her husband hit Subway—as long as he's mindful. "I've learned how to make it work for us. We can go, but let's get the chicken breast and chocolate milk instead of the huge super-combo or the 16-ounce soft drink," she says. It's all about moderation, as my Uncle Chet likes to say, and the same thing should hold for your next few weeks of training.

During Week 14, run twice for twenty-five minutes, and, if possible, do it without walking. A lot of people run their first 5K (3 miles) and then take a breather, and that breather becomes the end of their racing career. Don't do that. Sign up for your 10K. Pick something about three months away. In Week 15, add a third run to your training. Keep your first two consistent at twenty-five minutes, but on run number three, try and bump up the time you spend running to thirty-five minutes. Again, diet and training share many similarities. Both involve delaying gratification for some future reward.

Richard Simmons, among my all-time favorite interview subjects, is both a runner and a diet expert, and he had to learn the hard way about the dangers of doing anything in the extreme. "When I was a runner, I'd gone from 268 pounds to 119 pounds, but I did it by starving and throwing up," says Simmons, who everyone should have the good fortune to meet (twice during our interview he cried). "All we think about is how good that food's going to taste, then we eat it, and two hours later we hate ourselves. I had to make a plan—you can't eat healthy without a plan."

ARE YOU writing down the results of your runs? If you also write down what you're eating, you'll eat better, and less. According to Dr. James Painter, chairman of the School of Family and Consumer Sciences at Eastern Illinois University, the reason that dietician Nicole Yuen can eat well is that she's not oblivious to food; she's paying attention. Every time she walks into a 7-Eleven, she doesn't feel threatened because she knows what the food that she eats does to her. Thinking about nutrition choices is part of her routine.

"Anything we do for a short period of time fails; the only things that last are legitimate lifestyle changes," says Painter, who, like all of our nutrition experts, stresses that it's not about giving up provolone cheese, barbecued meats, or vodka but moderating your intake and making bad foods (or fatty foods or caffeinated drinks or candy) a treat for once in a while. The point isn't to binge and purge like I do (though less often now), but to make small changes that will hold over time.

"I probably ate too much junk food all my life. If I traveled to a hotel, I'd order up a plate of nachos with cheese and I was big with Doritos," says Bill Rodgers, the last American-born citizen to win the Boston Marathon, a race he won four times. "Back then, we didn't know what we know now about nutrition, but also I was hungry."

If you're running three times a week, General Tso's chicken won't kill you. And while Julie's pregnant and craving McDonald's, I'm not going to be the schmuck telling her I can't have one of her french fries. You have to celebrate your hard work.

"I always celebrated," says Rodgers. "I'd have a gin and tonic, or two, or three, after a big race and order up my favorite meal, which might be a cheeseburger. You have to celebrate in this sport. It's hard."

THE SOUNDTRACK: Kendrick Lamar

My nephews started listening to rap music and it was all the cartoon stuff: Flo Rida, Two Chainz, Soulja Boy, whatever else was on the radio and in their school hallways. They were learning it wrong. Kendrick Lamar's record is different; remorseful, it has second thoughts. Life isn't a party and gangsta stuff isn't cool, and though he's from Compton, California, Lamar introduced something new to hip hop, or at least something my nephews had been missing: nuance.

This book was finished when I interviewed him and I had basically moved off music to work on my running stuff full-time. No matter. I had to thank Kendrick in person. I wanted him to autograph my nephews' CD. Jakob and Dimitri, these are the running songs that he recommends.

"Let's Fall in Love," The Isley Brothers: "On this day, you're jogging, but not only exercising, you're having peace of mind. This song is for your time to do you. You may have kids, you may have a job, things that totally consume you, but when you hear this one, take some time for self-reflection on who you are. It's for a little alone time with yourself, yup."

"Against All Odds," 2Pac: "To get your juices flowing, 2Pac. This is on your energetic day—you're really pumped up and excited. You have goals ahead, something through the week that you want to tackle. When you want to stay focused and have that energy, you play this record right here."

8

I FEEL BAD ABOUT
MY SPLIT TIMES

THE TRAINING: Speed Work, Works

WEEK 16: Run once this week for 21 minutes, once for 25 minutes, and once for 37 minutes. During the 21-minute run, run like mad for a minute at the 5-minute, 10-minute, 15-minute, and 20-minute marks.

WEEK 17: Run twice this week for 25 minutes and once for 39 minutes.

THE SOUNDTRACK: Ben Gibbard

THE FINISH LINE: The 10K race, now 11 weeks away.

THERE ARE two ways to go running. Both are good, but one's certainly better, especially if you don't want to just finish but actually get faster with each race. At some point, it's not enough just to run the same lazy circle around your block. Running's monotonous? Run faster. Try harder. Risk more. Although you can increase your endurance by running incrementally longer distances and gradually weaning yourself a minute at a time from walking, you will eventually have to bring the crazy: allow yourself the freedom to go as fast as you can.

"I'm at the point where I want to improve and not feel like a beginner," says Reena Basser, a mother of three, who sent me an email not long ago. Since Basser lives close to a deli I like, and I know Julie's always up for chopped liver, I pay her a house call and check out her routine. Even though she's a regular runner, getting out as much as six times a week, her workout never changes. It's the same forty-five-minute loop of walking and running each time. Since she's never signed up for any races, she's never altered her level of effort, and that's why today she's feeling stuck.

"I looked at some running blogs, but they're not encouraging. One said, 'If you're going to run a ten-minute mile, it's better to jump into a pool of ice cream,'" Basser says. So we went out to a park in front of her house and tried something different. Instead of running ten laps slowly, as she does every day, we added a thirty-second dash to the end of each loop. Basser wears a long skirt and long sleeves with her New Balance sneakers; she doesn't look like a track star. But so help me God, I saw this Orthodox Jewish woman transform into Mary Keitany. "Wow, that's fun. That's exciting!" she says, after she's finished her first little sprint, out of breath and ready to try it again. "You see yourself in a different way. You're not this slow, plodding fat person who can't do anything—you feel like you actually have speed."

YOU'RE RUNNING three times this week, twice for something like twenty-five minutes and once for about ten minutes longer—this is your introduction to the long run. The long run will be the cornerstone of your training and probably the single most important exercise you'll do between now and the marathon. You can skip one of these twenty-five-minute runs and survive 10K (6 miles). These runs are for building strength, working on your stride, and accumulating miles in your legs. In the world of dining, they're akin to eating lunch at your desk while you work: not glamorous, but important—after all, you gotta eat. But the long run is different. It's Friday night on the town. If you're running alone, it might be smart to start carrying a few dollars. Nothing's worse than getting stuck forty-five minutes from your house with no scratch for the bus.

It just makes sense that things become more fun as you get better at them, though it takes time. Kate Hays, a sports psychologist who was in charge of the New York City Marathon's Psych Team and now works with the GoodLife Fitness Toronto Marathon, told me this is called "mastery"; as you become more skillful, your task becomes more pleasurable, you do it more, you get better faster, and you create a positive feedback loop. This week, we introduce a few running drills that might speed up your mastery of the sport. If you feel up to it, at five, ten, fifteen, and twenty minutes into your twenty-five-minute run, add a twenty-five-second dash. These dashes are called fartleks—they're what I ran with Reena Basser—and they'll make you faster. However, be wary. Don't go so quickly at five and ten minutes that you have no hope of completing your run. To "win" this drill, first of all you have to finish; second, the last dash should be as quick as the first one. Figure out what feels right to you. See what you're doing? Exactly what I don't do when it comes to remodeling the bathroom: getting involved.

The long run is still the priority, so if you're challenged enough by the regular training—in which we endeavor to run up to nearly forty minutes—forget about this other stuff. In your marathon training it's more important to build distance than speed. But, if you're hungry to work in little challenges, try this: in Week 17, instead of one of your twenty-five-minute runs, find a decent-sized hill that you can run up and down, and do it three or four times. This exercise will also help you with your form. Of course, it's goofy. You will look funny going up and down the streets in fluorescent shoes, especially when schoolchildren are beside you, with their sleds. But races are held on all kinds of terrain, and even if your only goal is to finish, why not finish prepared? Hill training is great for building strength in your legs and core, and by diversifying your workouts your interest remains high. It takes more effort to run up a hill than to jog for twenty-five minutes on a treadmill. Think about that when you envision yourself crossing your 10K finish line. You won't be bored.

THE CANADIAN record in the marathon was set by Jerome Drayton in 1975, which is a hell of a long time ago for a record to hold. However, if it were broken tomorrow, many of us would guess that it was snapped by Reid Coolsaet, the first Canadian male to qualify for the London Olympics and a friend of mine who was previously introduced rather unceremoniously for having to take a crap in the middle of a race. Coolsaet deserves better; he's not only one of Canada's fastest marathoners but its most consistent—even though in his freshman year at the University of Guelph he didn't make his cross-country team. "I thought people were better runners than me because of genetics more than anything else. I didn't understand how much training actually mattered," says Coolsaet, who credits his remarkable improvement to a combination of increased mileage, attention to nutrition and core strength, training in Kenya, and running with a team that also includes Eric Gillis, who won the Vancouver Sun Run in 2011 (and would later join him on Canada's 2012 Olympic marathon team). "So many things in life are about instant gratification, but in running, there's not really any shortcuts. It's something that takes a long time to get good at."

Clearly, if you hate running, it's going to be difficult to put in the necessary mileage to improve. Someone who busts out a few fartleks on a run after dinner is not someone cursing their every step. Coolsaet points out that if you look at the world's best runners, like Jamaican sprinter Usain Bolt, they usually have a smile on their face. Sometimes you should try to do more than just put another red X for a completed workout on your calendar. You know how long the loop around your house is. On today's run, why not try and do it two minutes faster?

Push yourself in practice and you won't have to push yourself quite so hard in the race. The Kenyan motto? Train hard, win easy.

"PEOPLE WHO don't do anything can do a marathon; it just comes down to willpower," says Richard Lee, a distance coach in Vancouver who trained his first runner in 1984, taking his wife, Sue, all the way to the Olympics in Los Angeles. "You're not born with talent one way or the other—it's a learned process. You just need to be prepared, set and follow a plan, and develop a steel-trap mind for achieving your goals."

Matt Loiselle, a Canadian marathoner who competes with Reid Coolsaet, turned me on to a new training method, and I really like it. Once I even did it in the rain. I try to run one mile six times, all of them under six minutes. The goal is to complete the sixth mile as quickly as the first. I do this down by the lake, where there are no stoplights, and if you saw me, cursing and sprinting and psyching myself up, you'd think I was nuts. Kids point and laugh. But this kind of running isn't monotonous. We're not made out of sugar. We don't melt in the rain and it's OK to push. Running should hurt sometimes. Doesn't love?

"ANY TIME we're making a commitment, we're making a choice to give up other choices. But we're so inundated with messages throughout the culture not to give up anything that sometimes we feel like we're making a mistake," says Scott Stanley, co-director of the Center for Marital and Family Studies at the University of Denver and author of *The Power of Commitment*. Stanley talks a lot about the dangers of "half-commitments" and the difference between sliding and choosing. Mastery, Hays told me, is about overcoming indecision and committing to something, full stop. It's better to get married or break up than to spend ten years trying to decide whether or not to get a ring.

With running, it's the same thing. If you follow a program and punch a clock, mindlessly doing the same thing every day, you won't reach your potential. The beauty of the long run and speed work is they help you take ownership of your progress. Tweak, plot, plan—mix things up, fail a few times, participate in the sport. "Inertia, in terms of running, is where people get caught up in the excitement, but haven't really decided yet that they're a runner. They're doing it, but maybe just sort of following along," says Stanley, a former runner who admits to slowly falling away from the sport. "The best way to fight inertia is through little incremental changes. You can't become a runner in a day, just like you can't improve your marriage in a morning, but you can take little steps toward owning whatever it is that you're after. In a marriage, it's not about jumping on a hand grenade, it's about waking up early to clean the stove."

Inertia can affect runners whose running doesn't change. You run the same boring loop in the same boring time, and you're coasting. It's like staying at a job for too long. You're half-in and half-out. Speed work's an antidote to the tedium. So on one of your runs this week, try to find your own version of my six-times-one-mile madman. Even thirty seconds of running quickly on a twenty-five-minute run will help make you fast. Every time I run I know exactly how much effort I'm expending, and this gambit usually plays itself out at yellow lights. You shouldn't stop every time.

HERE'S ONE more story, from Betty Lee, who went from the couch to the marathon in only one year: "I hated running. I thought it was waste of time," says Lee, a self-employed financial analyst in Toronto, who used to describe her body as pear shaped but realized that, over time, it had begun to look more like an apple. "Even after I lost twenty kilograms, I thought running was going to kill me; but after a few weeks, I wanted to go a little farther—I had that energy." Lee began her first Learn to Run clinic at the Running Room in May 2010, and in May 2011 she finished the GoodLife Fitness Toronto Marathon. Her progress is extraordinary for just how normal she is. It was a sedentary lifestyle and McDonald's french fries that drove her to running, and during her training she took time off between November and January because, like most people, she couldn't stand running in the cold.

"I looked at myself and saw that I'd begun to carry the fat in my midsection, and it got me thinking this is not good," says Lee, who modified her diet to keep in shape for the gradually increasing distances in her running clinics and augmented her running workouts with boot camp classes twice a week.

"We tend to talk ourselves out of something, but if you keep those negative thoughts at bay, running can get in your blood." Betty Lee didn't set out to run a marathon in her first year as a runner, but she enjoyed her clinics and kept pushing her goal a little farther. When she started, she knew she sucked and she didn't like it, and so she asked questions of runners she passed in the park and during her running classes. Eventually, she adapted her stride so that she didn't land so much on her heel.

Pay attention to how you're running. It will both make the running more fun—being cognizant of what you're doing gets you more involved—and make your training an active process. Now when Lee runs she's careful to land on the balls of her feet, barefoot style, not on her heels. You want to sound less like an elephant, someone told her, and more like a deer. Think about what you need to do to get more from your running. If you want to go faster, you need to spend some time doing drills. Pay attention to lifting your knees when you feel yourself getting tired, and remember to look in the direction where you want to be. Watch any race. The people who stop are the ones looking down.

In my last prenatal course, the nurse was talking about caring for the baby during the first forty-eight hours. She kept saying: don't miss the cues. In how many other instances is that advice appropriate?

Don't miss the cues and you won't get injured.

Don't miss the cues and you won't slowly become slower, until you're a fraction of the runner you used to be.

Don't miss the cues and you won't feel guilty when you head out of town for a run.

Don't miss the cues. I guess that, more than anything, is how you finish the race.

THE SOUNDTRACK: Ben Gibbard

Ben Gibbard, the lead singer of The Postal Service and Death Cab for Cutie, ran the LA Marathon in 2011 in 3:56:34. Gibbard's a hero of mine because he came to running after giving up drinking and is candid in talking about how he transformed: "One of the side effects of being a musician is every night that you play a show you're providing your audience with a Friday night," Gibbard says. "It's easy to get into the mindset that, since it's their Friday night, it's our Friday night too." The Postal Service had been retired, and Gibbard had a year off from Death Cab, and during this time he blacked out at a buddy's house in Big Sur. It's a hazard that comes with his job. "Normal people don't drink at work and go drinking after work five nights a week, but as a touring musician it can become your expected behavior," he says. "I got carried away and took it back home."

Gibbard never ran as a kid, but he got to the marathon in a four-month program—during which time he also quit booze—and today, even though he's split from what's-her-name, he's still running and finding inspiration in Haruki Murakami's book *What I Talk about When I Talk about Running*. I love that after his marriage broke up, Gibbard reunited The Postal Service and began playing stadiums again. He says he burned through thousands of songs during his training and had his music set up into playlists: Run I and Run II. These are the highlights of the mix:

This Is Happening, LCD Soundsystem: "Someone gave me this, and I've listened to it at least one hundred times while I'm running. It seems to just have the right beats per minute, but there's also an attitude lurking beneath the dance tracks. It almost has an old-school flavor, but it sounds totally crisp."

"Burning Inside," Ministry: "That shit was like my aggro jams from high school. No matter how much new stuff is out there, you always kind of come back to the stuff that influenced you when you were young. Love Ministry, love them."

"My Mathematical Mind," Spoon: "Britt, the lead singer, is a friend of mine and a runner too and I always ask him if he wrote this song while running: the BPMs are lined up just right. Whenever this comes on, I get in a zone."

9

HOW THE
BODY WORKS

THE TRAINING: Creeping Above 40 Minutes

WEEK 18: Run 3 times this week, once fast for 20 minutes, once at average speed for 30 minutes, and once slowly for 40 minutes, covering more ground. This is your long run.

WEEK 19: Again, run 3 times: 25 minutes; 35 minutes; and then, instead of the long run, speed work or hills.

THE SOUNDTRACK: Lionel Richie

THE FINISH LINE: Nine weeks before the big 10K.

THIS WEEK, build on the drills you began last chapter. Can you feel yourself getting stronger? Keep writing down the results. Think of this log as a growth chart for your talent. Be prepared to spend more than an hour on your feet during your 10K (6-mile) race. And the only way to get ready for that is to try it first in practice.

Last week's long run should've topped out at about forty minutes, which is awesome. If you can run forty, you can run sixty. It's easier to put the pedal to the metal when strangers are cheering, traffic's stopped, and you're running alongside, say, 60,000 people at the Peachtree Road Race in Atlanta. It's much harder running by yourself on a cold February morning before work. This week, stay with the three workouts and add two minutes to your long run, creeping above forty minutes and learning to adjust your pace to greater distances. If you didn't get up to forty minutes last week, fine. Just add two minutes to whatever you did. But you're coming up on nineteen weeks of running. And if you've been keeping up—even just approximating your runs—you should feel confident: the 5K's done, here comes the 10.

Next week, keep two of your runs consistent at twenty-five minutes and experiment with the third. If you did fartleks last week, this week try running 1,600, 1,200, 800, 400, and 200 meters (1 mile, 1,300 yards, 875 yards, 435 yards, and 220 yards), twice, making sure your second set of intervals is as fast as the first. Or, if you'd prefer, try hill runs. The important thing is to keep tweaking your workouts because you want to work different muscles when you train. When running hills, you naturally lift your knees, keep your back straight, and land on your midfoot. You'll fall down if you land on your heel. So find a place near your home with some vertical. It doesn't have to be a ski slope. The hill I run takes me two minutes to climb, and I do it eight or ten times. Do this once a week, or every third week, rotating in speed work and long runs, and you'll have extra kick in your final kilometer as you race 10K.

I DIDN'T RUN today. Julie and I had a daughter: Esme Marrietta Kaplan, born August 20, a half-Peking Duck–sized ball of lungs and fur and triangle ears and two specs of gorgeous beige eyes. It was an emotional evening: I cut the umbilical cord and counted the fingers and toes, but Julie did most of the work. Now I'm watching over my girls, both of them sleeping, and I'm moved, drunk with emotion and coaching an eight-hour battle, awed—standing at the starting line and the finish line at the same time. Lord, give us strength, or a peppermint schnapps and a sandwich. Make Julie and me like our mothers and fathers . . .

Little Esme, good morning. We're your parents. There's nothing, for you, we won't do.

NOW LET'S TALK about what happens to the body when we run. Think of the right and left sides of the body as two springs. When we run, we just bounce along the avenue, transferring energy from one body part to the next, moving in a kind of unconscious symphony that grows more powerful over time. It seems counterintuitive to be relaxed while running, but the body does that naturally: while one side's working, the other's preparing for its turn. Running is basically hopping: even when running ultramarathons, the distance is covered one leg at a time. In other words, running is a series of one-legged motions. Only when we stop running do we have both feet on the ground. So how do we hop? Well, to create energy, the body burns oxygen, and as we run, we increase our breathing, meaning our lungs are working just as hard as our heart. Our lungs are as important as our legs.

Energy gets the body in motion: the heart pumps blood, the blood flows to the muscles, the muscles contract and expand, and we move forward. It's a beautiful thing—our heartbeat is like Flea, that marathon runner from the Red Hot Chili Peppers; it creates the bass line—and the best part is we don't need to think about any of this stuff; it just happens. But if we can learn a thing or two about how the body works—why our knees ache and why sitting affects the flexibility in our

hips*—we can help stave off injury and feel a little more connected to our joints and arteries as we put them through hell.

"The more oxygen you take in, the more energy you create,
the faster you run," says Dr. Greg Wells, a scientist and physiologist at the University of Toronto and author of the book
Superbodies. "When we run, the body increases the produc-
tion of mitochondria—our own natural form of energy—and
we can transform our internal engine from a V4 to a V8. It's
the way we become turbo-charged." Internally, the body
transfers its energy. Externally, we move through two phases
with each stride: the swing phase and the return phase—
basically, when we kick out and when we bring the leg back
in. For the swing phase, the quadriceps muscle extends the
leg and the hamstrings help balance our hips. Since most of
our running power extends from the hips, think of the leg as
Indiana Jones's bullwhip. The whip snaps at the hip joint, but
the ankle and knee also move from that initial motion. Everything's connected. If our bodies were a TV show, they'd be
The Wire.

In each leg, a series of muscles move in harmony, transferring energy from the toes through the lower leg up the thigh
through the ass and into the back and spinal cord. The trans-
ference of energy spreads through our body like a crowd at a
baseball game doing the wave. When the knee is perpendicu-
lar to the ground, at the apex of our stride, we move from the
swing phase to the return phase. So, as the oxygen pumps
through our veins, building red blood cells and transferring
energy to our muscles, the hips, feet, and lower leg begin their
continuous cycle. When the blood starts pumping, we take in
more oxygen, and as we keep breaking down and rebuilding
our muscles, we find that, even at rest, we have more energy:
welcome to the feeling of being in shape.

"You'll feel horrible in the first few weeks of becoming a runner, because the body's not used to the initial burst of stress, but the oxygen transport pathway of the body can be strengthened, and when this happens, you're improving your overall health," says Dr. Wells, himself a runner and an extreme cyclist, who once rode his bike 11,000 kilometers (more than 6,800 miles) across Africa. "Before you look good on the outside, on the inside, your body's already getting in shape."

We've talked about how our bodies have evolved since the Stone Age to help us run: our toes are short, our head generally sits well balanced on our neck, our tendons are springy, our glands produce sweat, and our bodies are relatively hairless (at least compared with baboons). Think there's no way you can run 10K? Imagine that you've already spent three million years, genetically speaking, getting ready for your chance. For once, think about the Achilles tendon, the bit that attaches the calf to the heel. It provides elastic energy, which we use when we run. Elastic energy works in the legs like a spring—we push down and bounce up like a coil. In that sense, we are our own energy-generating trampolines. And creating this power source gets easier the more you do it, especially as you get lighter.

How we run is simple: the skeleton holds us together, oxygen gives us fuel, and the Achilles tendon transfers energy to our legs. "You can walk without a long Achilles tendon, but you need the Achilles tendon for the elastic return of a run," says Dr. Irene Sprague Davis, the Harvard professor in charge of the Spaulding National Running Center and one of those nuts who runs without shoes. Davis is a proponent of the evolutionary theory of running. Like her colleague Daniel Lieberman's studies, Davis's research indicates that we have muscles in our feet that atrophy inside a heavily cushioned running shoe. If we want to run without being injured, she believes we should maximize the inherent strengths in our physiology.

"There's no indication that we've really gained anything by the advent of these fancy shoes," she says, adding that muscle fibers, which are stored in our tendons, are released as we move, while the muscles expand and contract. The ankles flex, the knees flex, and under a load of tension, the muscles elongate, and that propels us forward. "Energy absorption becomes power generation, and you stretch like a rubber band when you move forward," says Davis. "Think of the muscles as a fist; they open and close as you go."

When we run, we engage our muscles and organs and we use our legs and arms, hips, head, and heart. Our arms swing forward to help drive momentum, our lungs take in oxygen, and our legs carry us across the finish line—we use our entire body when we use our legs.

DANA MURCHISON is a molecular biologist and works as a staff scientist at Science North, a museum in Sudbury, Ontario, which Canadians know is Alex Trebek's birthplace. Murchison was recently in charge of the popular *Body Worlds* exhibit and has a history of teaching science to kids. She's also training for her first 10K. Since how we run is simple, but explaining the mechanics behind it gets complicated, I asked her to tell me how the body works as if she were talking to a fourthgrader. "When you start to run, the body burns the energy that's already stored in the muscles. But once that's gone— and it only lasts for about ten or twenty seconds—your body regenerates energy and produces lactic acid," Murchison says. "Ever feel a burning sensation in your muscles? That's the body making lactic acid."

Once the body starts producing lactic acid, the workout triggers your anaerobic system, which kicks in once the cells have used up all the oxygen. See, as long as you're using oxygen as fuel, it's an aerobic workout. But when you exercise for a long time, you use up all that oxygen in your cells, and the workout becomes anaerobic because the body needs to find an alternative source of fuel. So we make lactic acid. "As you build up your training, your muscles develop, but so do your cardiac and respiratory functions," says Murchison, adding that everything improves while you train: your circulation, your ability to move oxygen in and out of your lungs, your aerobic threshold (how long you can work out before producing lactic acid), and even your cardiac strength (the heart is, of course, the body's most important muscle). "Your heart gets stronger as you train; that's why so much of postcardiac treatment relies upon exercise," she says. "It beats more, and with each beat it pumps more blood. This is why high-performing athletes have low resting heart rates: their hearts pump more blood."

WHEN WE run, each time we land, the force of impact can be as much as two-and-a-half times our body weight. That's called "loading," as in loading up all our weight on one joint at a time. The knees are the body's largest joint, and it's a hell of a crash landing they're forced to absorb. When we stand still, each leg supports half of our body weight. But when we run, since we land one leg at time, that's almost three times our body weight coming down with every step. That can be brutal, especially if we haven't completely felt all the effects yet of our new healthy eating. "The load's applied through the muscular and skeletal system through the body, but it's still a lot to be distributed across one leg," says Dr. John Challis, graduate school program director of kinesiology at Penn State University.

Our bones may be brittle, but they work like the heart or any other muscle—they get stronger as we train, and weight-bearing exercise can improve the body's bone-mineral density. Osteoporosis affects more than half of North Americans over the age of fifty, and of this group, 80 percent are women. In that sense, we run not only for what marathon training does for us now but what it will do in our glory years. (And if you're in your glory years now and training, welcome; I hope you like Ghostface Killah's musical recommendations.) In essence, we're strengthening ourselves today to stave off our eventual demise. "Loading develops healthy bones. In our mature years, loading maintains density and fights off the effects of old age," says Dr. Challis, who has written in the *Journal of Biomechanics* about how the body changes when we age. "People complain about how running leaves their knees or hips aching, but if standing still was sufficient loading, we wouldn't see half the population suffer from osteoporosis."

Whether or not we've evolved to arrive en masse at our local Starbucks before a race doesn't matter. The point is that complicated systems are at work in our bodies each time we run, and neurologically, physiologically, and endoskeletally most of us should be able to handle the shock to our system of a forty-five-minute run. Running makes our bodies grow stronger, and we tend to run in the way that unconsciously feels most natural. However you're running, do that.

* Our knees ache when we run because the quadriceps is actually a group of four muscles and sometimes each of those muscles isn't equally strong. This imbalance can wreck havoc on kneecap alignment. Sitting affects hip flexibility because that

motion weakens the glutes and shortens the hip flexors, the muscles we use to move our thighs.

THE SOUNDTRACK: Lionel Richie

Lionel Richie bugged me when we first met. He was two hours late, and then, when he arrived with his three assistants, one of them tried to order his lunch and he changed everything that could come with a plate of chicken breast over rice. I'm thinking, This asshole's daughter invented reality TV. Still, Lionel Richie! The guy started The Commodores, wrote "We Are the World" with Michael Jackson, and sold twenty million copies of "Can't Slow Down"—and what a great running anthem that is. He's probably earned the right to eat whatever he wants to.

Richie's also a runner and he told me he relies on the sport to help him change his mindset. "When I'm running, I see the world differently," he says. "It's like there's a fog, but when I get out there, the fog opens up."

He picked one song, his favorite running song of all time.

"Stairway to Heaven," Led Zeppelin: "When a black guy makes something that reflects his influences, it's called R&B; when a white guy plays R&B, they call it rock 'n' roll," he says, adding that, when running, he wants to listen to something with guitar and live drums. "When most people run, they have to move to a rhythm or the pace of a song, but I'm the other way around. I can have an acoustic guitar playing, and it puts me into a different mindset, when life was another way." Richie listens to Johnny Cash, Cream, and Marvin Gaye when he runs but declares "Stairway to Heaven" his all-time favorite tune: "It changes and keeps going—it has no restrictions and keeps opening up. When I'm running through the prism of that music, like the song, I feel like I can keep going for days."

10

ON ASSEMBLING
THE PERFECT
RACE OUTFIT

THE TRAINING: Shooting a 45

WEEK 20: Run for 30 minutes twice this week, and run once doing either speed work or hills.

WEEK 21: Twice this week, run for 25 minutes, but the big thing now is one long 45-minute run (walk, as ever, where needed).

THE SOUNDTRACK: Dolly Parton

THE FINISH LINE: The 10K, now just about 7 weeks away.

YOU'RE NOW able to run for so long that if you called Domino's and ordered a pizza, if it hadn't arrived by the time you returned, you'd be eating that pizza for free. This month, the long runs should top out around forty-five minutes. If you know how far you're running and how long it takes you, you'll be able to project your finishing time and make a time goal. If the goal is to finish, beautiful, focus on that. But if the goal is to finish, say, in fewer minutes than your age, then get a sense in practice of how fast you are. Don't make up an arbitrary goal: that's the stuff that will make you hate running. Instead, figure out how many kilometers your forty-five-minute loop is. Taking that number, figure out your average pace.

This week, again run three times, keeping the first and second runs consistent, something like thirty minutes. Then do a third run of either speed work or hills. After that, boost your long run. Set it up with a couple of runs for twenty-five minutes to keep your legs fresh, because you don't want to be out of practice when you try your forty-five-minute long run over the weekend.

Here's some basic information about the 10K: the average female finisher takes sixty-four minutes (and is thirty-five years old). The average male finisher takes fifty-five minutes and is thirty-seven years old. These statistics should give you some perspective about your own running. Now enough about all this "running," let's talk about clothes.

BETTY LEE doesn't like her butt, so when she runs, she wears a skirt. It's a little black number made with Lycra, polyester, and a sweat-wicking super-fabric, attached to a built-in pair of mesh underwear. "I don't like anything tight on my butt showing," Lee tells me, and she's no dilettante runner. Like I said, she went from her couch to completing a marathon in only one year. "I can run for three, four, five hours—but only if I'm in a skirt."

If you've made it this far without buying a whole heap of products, hallelujah—that's a feat almost as impressive as completing the marathon. But now, seven weeks away from your 10K, you're eating well and regularly running three times a week, and perhaps even mixing in some speed work and hills with your long run. It's time to wear spandex clothes.

Self-consciousness is a son of a bitch when you're running, so the stuff you wear should make you feel strong. Don't be mistaken. You can run beautifully without a $54 pair of pink Lululemon shorts with four-way stretch fabric that wicks moisture, but, at this stage of your training, you should have a few things to help make you feel comfortable. There's a reason this chapter is so far into your training: you've earned it.

I don't take spending money lightly. There's a cafeteria at the *National Post*, but I have no clue what the food is like. I may forget to buy pastries, but in five years I've never once forgotten to pack my lunch. Cash registers make me nervous, with reason. Julie and I once went to a sneaker outlet, and the sales guy—eager to help, knowledgeable . . . sorta, and just as friendly as can be—said, "You can wear these shoes for one marathon and then you have to throw them away." The guy was suggesting that a brand-new pair of sneakers was good for only up to five or six hours, as if they're some kind of chicken dinner that spoils if it's left out of the fridge.

Still, people who hate running generally are wearing the wrong things. When I went running with Rob Ford, he may have weighed 330 pounds, but he was probably carrying another ten pounds in soaking wet cotton. Running's totally natural, but doing anything for five hours is hard. It's a long time to sit on a couch. And while much is made of the Ethiopians and Kenyans who can run barefoot faster than someone in a new pair of $200 sneakers, know that whenever star African runners hook up with a sponsor, they forgo their days of running barefoot in blue jeans for the first tech-fit bra and polyester socks they can find.

In 2012, the most current year of the National Sporting Goods Association's statistics, running apparel purchases reached over $1 billion—with Garmin sports watches alone accounting for $322 million in sales. It was the biggest leap in any of the sportswear categories, which means runners buy and replace their crap more than swimmers, cyclists, gym rats, or any other weekend warriors. Mary Wittenberg, the organizer of the New York City Marathon, said her participants have an average household income of $130,000. There are plenty of places for them to park all that cash.

Like using it to buy socks. Cotton socks are no good for long distances, and in general you don't want any clothing—shirts, shorts, bras, capri pants—that absorbs moisture and bunches up. Ten kilometers can be grueling. In Ottawa, I felt like the distance between 6 and 7K (Miles 3 and 4) was about as far as running from Toronto to Barcelona.

In the summertime, you will sweat, and heavy fabrics will weigh you down. I wear synthetic socks that blend two types of polyester with a spandex band and that differentiate between my right and left foot. Does it matter if I put my left sock on my right foot? Probably not, but while at first the labels on my socks used to embarrass me, now I embrace them. (You know you're a runner when...) Similarly, other folks wear compression socks, nearly knee-high numbers that were designed to help diabetics with circulation. Listen, if they work for you, work it. Putting on funny clothing is part of the mental preparation. We're like knights suiting up for a battle. You can do a marathon in cotton gym socks. You can do one in army boots. But why?

"I FIND NEW runners don't want to wear clothes that look too technical, because they feel like they can't run fast. And there's a bit of embarrassment there, especially if they might be a bit of a bigger runner," says Jackie Turnbull, former design and development manager for Ronhill, an excellent British sports brand. (Hill, as in Ron Hill, is a former Olympic marathon runner and chemist who designed the first pair of running shorts with a slit on the side of the leg to allow better range of motion; he still consults on his company's clothes). "We know it's not just supermodels that run, and we want you to feel and look good. When you're starting, and beyond that actually, whatever you think suits you, that's the perfect running gear."

Stay away from spandex if you're self-conscious about your body. (And the same goes for neon.) If you're not in Arizona, wear black. It slims. Think about what you want from your outfit. Is it fashion first and then function, or the other way around? When you walk into the store, have a plan.

"When it comes to fluorescent and running, more is more," says Mosha Lundström Halbert, associate fashion director with Lord & Taylor, whom I take shopping one afternoon. I come out of the dressing room wearing black shorts with a black Ronhill tank top and my orange-and-yellow Adidas Bostons, and Halbert sends me back to the racks. "It's fine but nothing feels special, and since your sneakers are so bright, it feels like you're wearing a pair of Roots sweatpants with Louboutin shoes," says Halbert, herself a runner. We're joined by Betty Lee; Cory Freedman, founder of the Toronto Women's Runs series; Roger Moss, president of the Longboat Roadrunners and one of its coaches; Rahab Kamori, a non-runner who is visiting Toronto from Kenya; and Josphat Nzinga, her boyfriend from Eastern Kenya who has taken me under his wing. They all say that they choose clothes based on their ability to improve performance. But then they all comb the racks to pull together an outfit that looks sharp enough for a Saturday night (well, maybe in Boston during marathon week).

A lot of women run in three-quarter-length "capri" pants, which Halbert endorses, but I think men shouldn't wear pants that are cropped. When I'm racing, I like shorts with a zippered pocket, and preferably two. You probably already need to hold a house key—that's why shorts with a less secure Velcro pocket drive me nuts—and eventually you're going to want to pack energy gels (these are essential during the marathon). In general, and despite Halbert's warning, I feel shorts should be black, but go with what makes you feel good. She also warns against dressing too matchy-matchy—always a bad look.

A little fluorescent on my sneakers makes me feel fast, and if you get the same feeling from yellow short shorts, do your thing. Just make sure they're not falling off you. Even LL Cool J wears his shorts fitted snugly when he runs. Still, you don't want to look like you're dressing for a 1965 YMCA mixer. Make people wonder about the tippy-top of your leg. I love running shorts, but I don't wear them for anything other than running. If you're going to the beach, or having a casual day at the office, leave the spandex shorts at home.

"I feel like they're too short; I'll never wear these. They show too much lumpiness," Kamori says when she tries on a pair of snug blue shorts with a nice orange trim. Her boyfriend tells her the shorts look amazing, but the final decision is not his, and she ends up with a pair of plain black shorts with a black nylon liner that Halbert says look great.

Leigh-Anne Zavalick, product line manager for Saucony, who has the last word on all their men's and women's clothes, recalls reading an interview with *Sports Illustrated* swim-suit model Brooklyn Decker in which Decker was asked how she stays fit. Her answer was, in essence, that she doesn't wear clothing that hides her body. "Getting the body you want starts with being honest with yourself, addressing the reality, and by looking in the mirror and seeing what you actually look like," she says. Her comments bring to mind the premise behind keeping an eating and running log: the truth sometimes hurts, but the sooner you address it, the sooner it can change. "With running gear, the shorts and the Lycra, the fitted tops and exposed thighs, at least you know where you are."

All of your running clothes should feel comfortable. Don't buy anything that squeezes, pinches, or pulls. This stuff isn't Spanx and you're not Beyoncé; you're buying these clothes to work out. The clothes should fit snugly; you don't want air pockets and you don't want chafing and you don't want extra weight. But please, no suffocating. And for cold weather, think layering. The rule of thumb is to dress for the end of the race, not the starting line, as you heat up the longer you run. Everyone will find their own comfort zone in terms of dressing for weather. I asked Jessica Britton, the product designer of the Running Room, to give me five cold-weather dressing rules of thumb. Then I adjusted the list for my mom.

1. Over 10°C (50°F): shorts and a T-shirt
2. Around 4°C (40°F): tights and a T-shirt (or, what I prefer, shorts with a long-sleeved shirt; generally, I like to run in shorts when I can)
3. At –1°C (30°F): tights and a long-sleeved shirt
4. Near –9°C (15°F): tights, a long-sleeved shirt, and a vest (or some other three-garment variation that may or may not include armwarmers)
5. When the mercury hits –15°C (5°F): add a hat and gloves (although feel free to add these sooner)

REMEMBER, WHEN you're waiting for the bus, the air feels colder and the rain feels wetter than it does when you're running. And you can always take clothes off, but, once you're out there, you can't add. As with everything else, experiment. And add this information to your running log. Write down how you feel in what you run in, and then when the temperature hits, say, 4°C (40°F), you can flip through your little book to find out what you wore and how it felt.

I like running when it's freezing; Betty Lee does not. Don't get me wrong. I prefer running without a shirt on a beach in Hawaii, but for practical purposes, there's something about running in the cold that makes me feel like a tough guy. It's like actually using an SUV off-road. Every dentist's wife in Malibu is a jogger; you see them in spotless sneakers bouncing around the Santa Monica Pier. But only runners are out in February, in North Dakota, battling the ice and running through the snow. We spend plenty of time on the computer. Why not spend just as much time outdoors? This is the way to start to love running and see it become about more than just reaching 10K. Running through tough weather conditions can change how we see ourselves. Maybe I'm not as soft as I thought.

In the summer or early fall, it's a good idea to wear a dry-wicking shirt, which means the shirt's designed to pull perspiration away from your body. If you wear your shirt tight, your sweat won't have the chance to pool against your skin. When it's really hot, I like tank tops. Elite runners wear singlets, skinny tank tops that fit extra snugly. You don't want your shirt acting like a sail. If you're big, don't wear this type of top. Shirts are going to vary in thickness, which means that some are hotter than others, and there are also shirts that have pockets, zippers, and funny slogans. Don't wear shirts with funny slogans. And if you get a shirt in the goodies bag for your 10K, don't wear that shirt to the race. I know, I know, a lot of people do this. But it's like wearing a Dolly Parton shirt to a Dolly Parton concert. Maybe you can wear your Boston Marathon 2015 shirt to the Boston Marathon in 2039—that's hipster. But don't wear a race shirt to a race that you haven't yet run. It's unlucky. A race shirt must be earned.

"Running clothes can be tricky. I take cues from what's happening in fashion, but we also found that something like pastels, which are quite popular, don't feel fast, and designing running apparel's different than creating an Oscar gown," says Zavelick, the designer for Saucony. Her tips for first-time buyers? Don't buy oversized gear. Stay away from cotton. Find the color that best suits you, and the bigger-breasted you are, the more you need a good sports bra. Remember I mentioned fuming through a talk about sports bras at the Running Room the night before heading out to Ottawa to run my first race? Well, the guy's name is Vince Zamora, and he's been a Running Room manager for years. Obviously I didn't learn anything during his lecture, but I'm a reporter and I tracked him down.

How to Properly Shop for a Sports Bra: An Ode to Comfort, by Vince Zamora

1. Make sure there are no wrinkles and no bunching in the cup. If there's extra fabric, the bra's too big.
2. Place two fingers under the shoulder straps, one in the front and one in the back. If you can't slide your fingers under the straps, the bra's too small.
3. Don't be embarrassed to bounce around in the change room. Running's not a sedentary sport. How a bra fits sitting down isn't how it'll fit when you run.
4. Every time you buy a new pair of sneakers, buy a new running bra also. If your shoes are worn down, your bra probably is too.
5. Don't assume your regular bra and your sports bra are the same size. Try before you buy.
6. Your body's always changing, and what fit last year might not work anymore. Once again, try the bras on before you buy one.
7. Look for bras made with synthetic fabrics. Just like high-tech sportswear, your bra should keep you dry and comfortable.

Wear everything you're going to wear in your race first in practice; don't wear anything for the first time against the clock. Fit, size, color, material, fabric—all of these things boil down to personal preference: whatever makes you feel good is good. If you're self-conscious about your legs, try a black capri pant. Running at night? Wear a bright cap. And, most important, if you feel overwhelmed or confused, buy orange. This way, your friends will be able to pick you out in a race.

THE SOUNDTRACK: Dolly Parton

"I'm a very short little person with a big appetite," announces Dolly Parton, "and Lord knows, I've been up and down with my weight." Parton, a devotee of the Jane Fonda workouts, maintains a low-carb diet during the week then allows herself to enjoy whatever she wants on the weekends. Admittedly, it doesn't always turn out so great. "I lose weight, gain weight, and then go back on a diet again," she says. "I'm always on the job." Dolly Parton does squats and sit-ups, but she has also gone in for liposuction where she couldn't make Mother Nature bend to her whims. She's made forty-one records and is a savvy businesswoman beneath her backwoods Tennessee posturing. I interviewed her, lost the tape, and had to call her again. She gave me her running songs for a second time.

"In this business, they think you're a has-been if you're older than thirty-five. Me? I'm a little older than that," she says, "but don't forget the voice is also a muscle, and my voice is like a weightlifter—it just grows stronger after all these years." Dolly Parton isn't a runner, which is a shame, because she'd have insight to offer certain body types, but she's written 3,000 songs (including "I Will Always Love You," "9 to 5," and "Jolene") and was discovered by Johnny Cash at the Grand Ole Opry at the age of thirteen. These are her favorite groups and tunes:

The Louvin Brothers: "I love bluegrass music, and even though I sing all these different types of music, this is what's best suited for my voice. I don't listen to a lot of outside music, but when I need a shot of energy, I like putting The Louvin Brothers on."

"I'm Gonna Sleep with One Eye Open," Lester Flatt: "I love songs that give you a chuckle. How can that not make it easier getting through all that hard work?"

"I Can See Clearly Now," Johnny Nash: "Through the years that song's always been able to cheer me. I do like music that makes you feel good."

"Hitchin' a Ride," Vanity Fare: "Back in the day I used to listen to this song. It's just a great melody, great vocals, and a positive message."

"Everybody's Talkin'," Harry Nilsson: "Songs like that get your motor running."

THE BAD
STUFF

WEEK 22: Try 3 runs this week, each of them for 30 minutes, and see if you can continuously cover just a little bit more ground as you do so.

WEEK 23: This week, it's all about the long run. Go twice for about 30 minutes, then rest for a few days before attempting a 55-minute long run; however, please run slowly. If you can reach 1 hour, go for it, but look at the title of this chapter. The race is nearly upon us, and the most important thing is to not get hurt.

THE SOUNDTRACK: Marilyn Manson

THE FINISH LINE: The 10K, now just about 5 weeks away!

PEOPLE DIE running races. It happens all the time. And what happens to their bodies before they die is gruesome. A 10K race was held the other week in Toronto, and a nurse in the crowd stepped in to assist a runner who went down only a hundred meters from the finish line. "She had no pulse and she wasn't breathing," the nurse told a reporter at the *National Post*, where I work. "She was foaming at the mouth, and her eyes were rolled back."

That twenty-three-year-old girl is in the Intensive Care Unit of a hospital in Toronto, and I've been led to understand that, while on the mend, she's still in no condition to talk. I'm not even sure why I want to speak with her so badly, but I think it's because I want to know if she'd ever run a 10K again. Is it the running that did this? The medical results haven't been released yet, but it appears she suffered from cardiac arrest. And you hear similar stories all the time.

At the Chicago Marathon in 2011, a thirty-five-year-old firefighter named William Caviness from North Carolina collapsed 450 meters (about five hundred yards) from the finish line. He was pronounced dead less than two hours later. For one of the premier events in the world, it was the second fatality in five years. And when I ran the Toronto Marathon in May, Emma van Nostrand, aged eighteen, died of a heart abnormality, also just kilometers from the end of the race.

Is it irresponsible to send people to the marathon? Please, as you continue with your training, talk to your doctor. All of these runners thought they were healthy before the unthinkable happened; indeed, they probably thought they were in the best shape of their life.

If you can die in a 10K, what happens when you try to run four times that distance? "From the undertaker's perspective, driving an automobile is a much more dangerous endeavor than participating in a marathon," says Dr. Donald Redelmeier, Canada Research Chair in Medical Decision Sciences and the author of a study that looked at thirty years of American marathons. Studying a sample of more than three million runners, Redelmeier concluded that a city hosting a marathon

experiences 35 percent fewer fatalities on race day because of
the road closures. In other words, if you give the city streets
over to the runners, the city becomes safer because fewer people are in cars.

"The reason these running fatalities receive so much attention is that when someone drops dead in a marathon, you
think, Why didn't they just stay on the couch? The entire
situation could've been avoided, which is different from, say,
pancreatic cancer or Parkinson's disease, and while those
situations are plenty devastating, they don't attract the same
type of attention because these fatalities don't create the same
shock," says Dr. Redelmeier, who conducted his research,
published in the *British Medical Journal* in 2007, because he
was afraid that these types of horrific stories—stories of people foaming at the mouth with their eyes rolling back in their
heads—would scare people away from running.

Redelmeier has completed a marathon, and running, he
says, staves off diabetes, fights depression, and offers a host of
medical benefits, including strengthening the lungs, arteries,
and heart, which is why many post-cardiac arrest patients are
prescribed running as part of their recovery. "On any given
day, thousands of people exercise and thousands of people
don't quite exercise—thousands of individuals are right on
the threshold—and a small change in what your mother-in-
law or co-workers say can tip the balance toward inactivity
for thousands of people," Redelmeier tells me. "It's easy to feel
the shock of the deaths of these runners. They're evocative,
but misleading. Science provides evidence that for most of us,
running is better, not worse, for your health."

Here are the facts about cardiac arrest and running.
Between January 1, 2000, and May 31, 2010, in the United
States, there were fifty-nine cases of cardiac arrest in the

10.9 million marathon and half-marathon runners. In Canada, every seven minutes someone dies from heart disease or a stroke. In 2008, the population of Canada was right around 33 million. Of that group, 69,648 died of cardiac disease. It's not exactly apples to apples, but it certainly provides some perspective.

The problem is that running, like any strenuous activity, including sex, can exacerbate a pre-existing heart condition. What we generally see happening during races when runners go down is either a cardiac arrest or an exercise-related collapse. If it's just a collapse (and I don't mean to say "just" lightly; if you've seen someone go down during a race, it's a scary thing), it could be a result of low blood pressure or dehydration and generally doesn't require staying in a hospital overnight.

Cardiac arrest, however, can be deadly. Thankfully, the nurse resuscitated that twenty-three-year-old in Toronto, but of the fifty-nine race-related cardiac arrests suffered between 2000 and 2010, forty-two were fatal. Autopsies revealed, however, that well over 50 percent of the deaths occurred in runners who had already been suffering from a hardening of the arteries. The runners just didn't know it at the time. "The bottom line is, if you bring together any critical mass of people on any given day, there will be people in the crowd suffering from heart disease," says Dr. Aaron Baggish, associate director of the Cardiovascular Performance Program at Massachusetts General Hospital and the cardiologist for the Boston Marathon. "I've been running for twenty-five years—I'm a runner—and the only thing I worry about is getting slower. Running is one of the best ways to prevent cardiovascular problems."

Dr. Baggish conducted the study cited above for the *New England Journal of Medicine*, and for him, the interest in heart attacks among runners is personal. When he was just starting in medicine, he lost his best friend to sudden cardiac arrest. Nevertheless, Baggish runs. "You hear about someone dropping dead during a race and people say, 'Oh, these sports kill people, but that's not true; it's the opposite,'" says Dr. Baggish. "Running lowers your risk of dying and having a heart attack, but the paradox is if you do have a cardiac arrest—if you suffer from a pre-existing condition—that arrest is likely to happen while you exercise."

If you're following this training program, see your doctor. Run strenuously, but first, make sure that you can. If something's wrong, it's best to know now. In that way, running will already have saved your life.

This week, let's cool things down a bit with something like three thirty-minute runs. Last week, you had a long run and there's another one next week, so for now, just run easy and enjoy Dolly Parton's music selections. Maybe get a beer. Next week, run twice again for something like thirty minutes, and then shoot for a fifty-minute long run. On these journeys it's fine if you have to walk; what you want to fight against is giving up. In fact, walking for a minute every ten minutes might decrease your finishing time because it's better to walk once every ten minutes in a fifty-minute run than it is to run for thirty minutes and walk the entire last twenty minutes home.

As ever, life's all about pacing and I'm not doing so hot. Yesterday I ran, got home, and felt like I'd broken my back, which is bad because I'm five weeks away from running a marathon. If I finish the Scotiabank Toronto Waterfront Marathon in 3:10, I'll qualify for Boston. That hallowed race has an entry price— a qualifying time—you have to earn before you can even register to pay. Maybe, with the lack of sleep and the pressure of doing right by my wife and newborn, I should take a little something off each run. Instead I'm only going harder because I want a good time, and I'm beginning to think a lot about my Aunt Linda. When I told her I was running four times a week, expecting to impress her, she looked at me squarely and said instead, "What are you running away from?"

Running can be a great way to let off steam, but it can also become another source of frustration, addiction, stress. Right now I feel guilty taking all this time for myself. If the baby is jaundiced, should I not be doing mile repeats in the rain? My sister's having a difficult pregnancy in Denver, and Julie and I are about to take Esme to New York to meet my folks for the first time. That is, assuming they don't have to fly to Colorado and that we're not being idiots taking a one-month-old on a plane. I feel a little on edge. I told my best friend to fuck off and we've stopped talking, and between getting Esme's passport straight and the Diaper Genie working, it feels like each day takes five hundred hours. No wonder I'm limping around.

JANE CULLIS was three weeks away from running the Chicago Marathon when she felt a weird pain in her shin. A college varsity athlete, Cullis had run the half-marathon in 1:16 and was hoping to finish her second marathon somewhere around 2:40, which would make her one of the fastest marathon runners you'll meet, and more than thirty minutes quicker than me. "I was having one of the greatest buildups I'd ever had, reaching the highest mileage I've ever run, and feeling fitter than ever before in my life," says Cullis, who, at the time, was studying for her doctorate in medical biophysics.

Cullis had grown up dancing but was now running somewhere around 200 kilometers (130 miles) a week. Trained in science and a lifelong fitness junky, she began feeling indestructible, and so even though she was generally fatigued, she maintained her workout schedule before the marathon. "Two days before I was supposed to do my last big execution run, I felt a bit of soreness in my shin. I figured I'd be fine—I'd had soreness before and I'd run through it; it had never been anything serious—but I ignored what my body was telling me," says Cullis, who went out for her last 21 K (13-mile) run before the marathon and began to feel "a sharp, stabbing pain" in her shin. Again, she ignored the problem. This was her last hard run before her big race, and she figured she'd rest when she tapered before the marathon. "I felt like I had to get this last run in. I was hitting fast times and thought, I can't stop," she says, adding that when her final 21 K was finished and she had to jog home, she felt almost a crippling pain. It was as if someone were hitting her leg with a bat. After she made it home, she couldn't walk. And not only did Cullis not compete in the Chicago Marathon, but that was the last time she ran for a year.

"I'm not a reckless a person who wouldn't think about smart training, but you can get carried away," she says. "There's obviously a fine balance between the need for recovery and pushing your body, and I should've backed off. I felt the pain and ignored it. I went over that line." Cullis had strained her tendon, and then ignoring the problem, she tore it, making a small problem into a major issue and effectively curtailing a budding running career. Today she's a doctor, and after having an MRI done, she's once again running, and running fast through the streets of New York. But her story represents a significant concern that affects far more runners than a sudden heart attack: overuse.

"Most people, when they start out, they're so gung-ho that they do too much too soon," says Nicole Stevenson, one of Canada's all-time-fastest female marathoners and Cullis's former teammate and coach on the University of Toronto track team. "New runners just have to be careful because they'll face injuries right off the bat, like IT band syndrome, sore knees, and shin splints." Iliotibial, or IT, band syndrome affects the knee and results when the tissue extending from the pelvis to the knee gets inflamed, culminating in a stabbing sensation outside the kneecap. A good warm-up and cool-down of slow, easy running can help prevent it, as can wearing good shoes and stretching. Lying on your back, bring your left knee up to your shoulder and push your knee over to the right side of your body with your opposite hand, then switch sides.

Shin splints make up 15 percent of all running injuries. Too much mileage too soon causes shin splints, and these tiny breaks in the lower leg bones can be avoided, generally, by not increasing your mileage by any more than 10 percent in any one week.

It's good to push yourself—being tough is part of being a runner—but it's important not to be a dumb-ass. If you're doing speed work, warm up before and after you turn on the jets. If you feel tight, stretch. A good stretch for the hips is to get down on your hands and kick one foot back. Or stand up straight and lean from side to side, from the waist. If you feel pain in your quads, stand on one leg and bend the other, lifting it from your ankle.

When I went out to train with Reid Coolsaet and Eric Gillis, Canada's marathon stars, they hopped into a garbage can loaded with ice and cold water after their run. This cooling bath reduces soreness and promotes cell recovery to heal tiny tears in the muscle fibers. You may or may not do these things. I don't. But it's much more pleasant to avoid injury than recover from one.

"I find that for a distance runner, you have to be a patient person. You have to know your goal is months away, but train for it now," says Stevenson, who competed for Canada in the 2006 Commonwealth Games and ran the marathon in 2:32:56, setting a Canadian record. "Don't be a slave to your program. If something feels wrong, check it out. Runners tend to be obsessive people, but trying to squeeze in a run can sometimes do more harm than good."

The goal here isn't to freak you out but to encourage you to be smart: don't overdo it. And if you feel dizzy or as if you're going to faint or throw up or really anything other than just being plain old tired, please, listen to your body. Sometimes the best thing a runner can do is to stop.

THE SOUNDTRACK: Marilyn Manson

I very nearly got to fly out to L.A. to meet Marilyn Manson and interview him face to face. However, the music industry isn't doing so hot, and at the last minute, to my grave disappointment, we had to conduct the interview without Absinthe and over the phone. Still, Manson was awesome. "I ride a bike. I don't run because my feet are too big," Manson said, and when I asked how he's lived this long, he told me: "I sold my soul to the devil."

The truth is, Marilyn Manson is pretty funny. He gave us two running tunes.

"The Flowers of Evil," Marilyn Manson: "I recommend my own song and my own second verse: '*I've been running from the bloodless for fear of exile/for all of my sorceries that shun the light.*' It wasn't really written to describe a marathon, but lyrics are meant to be interpreted in different ways."

"Heading Out to the Highway," Judas Priest: "I don't listen to a lot of heavy stuff. I'm friends with Kerry King from Slayer, but when I listen to music I actually listen to a lot of mellow stuff—Gershwin, Bauhaus, The Beatles' *White Album*, Thelonious Monk. But if I really wanted to get wound up, I'd play, 'Heading Out to the Highway,' loudly, by Judas Priest. That's a good running song."

12

LETTER
FROM KENYA

THE TRAINING: Foot off the Gas

WEEK 24: Do 3 runs, for 30 minutes each, though use caution. If you're feeling tired, reduce the schedule to 2 runs this week. However, if you need to exorcise excitement, on 1 training run try fartleks for 30 seconds at 10-minute intervals.

WEEK 25: Taper, call your mother, and rest. Go out twice for about 25 minutes each and stay limber, but no speed work, no hills, no long runs. Don't overtrain. If the race is Sunday, enjoy your last run on Thursday. The important thing now is what you don't do.

THE SOUNDTRACK: Michael Bublé

THE FINISH LINE: The 10K, now just about 3 weeks away.

PREPARED FOR race day? Know what you're going to eat, where your socks are, how you're getting to the event? Keep the chores simple, reduce race-time decisions in advance, and taper until you get to the starting line. If your race is on Sunday, don't run after Thursday, and even that run should be slow and no more than twenty-five minutes long.

When you're two weeks away from your 10K, there's nothing wrong with a thirty- or even forty-minute jog. You can't make up for three months of training in an evening, but there's something comforting about knocking out the distance in practice before attempting it in a race. If you choose to do so, and you have to gauge this stuff for yourself, don't attempt it any later than nine days before race day. Don't train to train. Train to race.

I'M IN a hotel room with Robert Mwangi and Kenneth Mungara, the man with the fastest marathon time ever recorded on Canadian soil. We're watching television, and a commercial comes on. Sally Struthers is encouraging us to raise money for Africa, and we watch as flies buzz around the mouths of the kids in the ad. "This is what people here think of when they think of Africa," I tell them. They don't really respond, and we continue to chill. The commercial ends, and the show we're watching—*CSI* or some other cop show—comes back on and we watch as a drug dealer kills his rival before the police storm in and kill everyone. "This is what people in Africa think of the United States," says Mungara, and he smiles at his cousin.

I'd never known anyone from Africa before I got involved with running, but now I've met lots of people, mostly Kenyans and Ethiopians, and interviewed them and followed them around on jogs. They're the best runners in the world. The record time for finishing the marathon is 2:03:38, set by Patrick Makau at the Berlin Marathon in 2011. Makau is from Kenya, as is Sammy Wanjiru, who won the men's marathon gold in the 2008 Olympics in Beijing. At the London Olympics in 2012, Stephen Kiprotich, a runner from Uganda, took the marathon's gold medal, and second and third place fell to athletes who call Kenya home. At the Boston Marathon, 2013's winner, Lelisa Desisa, is Ethiopian; the women's winner, Rita

Jeptoo, is Kenyan, and the winners of the 2011 and 2012 men's marathon are Kenyan, too. The winner of the New York City Marathon in 2011 (because 2012 was canceled in the wake of Hurricane Sandy) was Geoffrey Mutai, who is Kenyan.

It's three days before the big race in Toronto, and Mungara is doing very little. He's won the last two Toronto marathons, and, even as a father of three and at thirty-seven years old, he likes his odds of picking up $20,000 for first place. Everything he does, he does slowly. While we're watching cop shows, I finish the cup of tea he gives me before he can locate the stir stick. He tells me the bath he took this morning was two hours long. If he's nervous about the race, he doesn't let on. And he laughs and shows me photographs of his daughters at a languid, countryside pace.

Technically, I'm competing in the same race as Mungara and his cousin, but they're tall and thin and from a place where you don't need Mayor Bloomberg warning of the dangers of the supersized soda. I'm probably not going to catch them, yet their approach to the sport is still an education. Not just in running, but in grace. "Ever walk somewhere with a Kenyan racer? You'll keep having to look behind you to see where they are," says Cliff Cunningham, the Toronto Marathon's athletic trainer in charge of wrangling elites from all over the world. It's about conserving energy, remaining coiled, being still, or moving slowly until the moment the racer needs to explode. "I want to listen to what's happening around me—even my own pain," says Mungara, who doesn't use energy gels, listen to an iPod, or even have a coach. "We all train and we all push, but the winner's the person who runs the smartest race."

THIRTY-FIVE SLEEPS after my daughter was born, I finally ran a smart race and finished beautifully in the half-marathon. I was thinking I might run only 1:40, as I'd been a ball of nerves all month, not sleeping, fighting with everyone, and hobbling around on one leg. But the day of the race the weather was perfect and I went out slowly and light, free of expectations and pressure, and I smiled.

After 3K (1 mile), I sped up and talked to everyone while I ran. That's the best. When a race isn't necessarily a "race," just a Sunday jog with people handing you cups of water and police keeping the traffic at bay. Sometimes I forget: running is fun. Not this time. And around halfway, I'd brought my split down to about 4:20-per-kilometer (6:58-per-mile) and felt like I still had more in the tank. My smile grew broader, and I sped up again and began passing people, feeling like I was on a rocket and everyone else was frozen in space. This race I was careful to take the energy gels being offered every few miles. I sang along to Joan Jett's "Bad Reputation." On this day, there was no limp, no rum, no anguish. I was just out there running around on a pretty Sunday, blasting away my make-believe adversaries like a juvenile delinquent going after ants with a magnifying glass. I came in at 1:29:55, exhausted, but in a good way—exalted, having left everything behind on the course. I had run the vaunted negative split. I'd run previous half-marathons faster, but I didn't enjoy them as much.

Keep this in mind on race day: give yourself realistic goals, perhaps just to finish. And spend as much time taking in the experience as you do fighting it. I don't always do this. But when I do, I love to run. This is something I've taken from Kenya. Wesley Korir, who won the Boston Marathon in 2012, once told me he doesn't pray for his races; he races to pray. And when Gilbert Kiptoo was in Vancouver for the marathon, he received a phone call—back home in Kenya his father had died. Kiptoo was in a strange country, barely spoke the language, hated the food, and missed his mother. He relaxed once during that week in Canada, when he ran the Vancouver

Marathon in 2:27 and came in fourth. That's when he *relaxed*. It's hard to run 10K when you're clenched. And that's what you can take from the Kenyans and use in your race.

What else? My friend Josphat Nzinga, who's from Kathiani, Kenya, east of Nairobi, ran barefoot 10K to and from school every day as a boy. Kenya's mountainous and has a higher elevation than Denver, and because these guys have grown up training on such difficult terrain, even something like Heartbreak Hill at the Boston Marathon doesn't seem so bad. You may not have grown up running as much as Nzinga, but that's why running hills should be part of your training. Most races aren't flat. And they're rarely called because of weather. Nzinga couldn't just skip school if it rained, so he got used to running in the elements, which is important. Don't skip a day if it's hot or cold or snowing or if you have a stuffy nose or the baby has an earache. Get used to running under less-than-perfect conditions now and you'll be able to handle them later on. But let your training slide just a little and your fitness, your motivation, your running program, all of them, fall apart. At least that's what I'm afraid will happen to me.

And another thing: Josphat Nzinga's diet is at least 26.2 times better than mine. In Toronto, he subsists on cooked meat, greens, fruit, milk, and ugali, a porridge-type stew made from water and maize—a complex carbohydrate that's loaded with starch. And Wesley Korir may spend half the year in Ontario, but you're not going to see him at the Dakota Tavern at two in the morning, three sheets to the wind and waiting for Kevin Drew to show up. Furthermore, Kenneth Mungara has never had a beer, smoked pot, or even puffed on a cigarette—stuff I did five nights ago, just eight days from my marathon, when Julie and I went see Feist (on Yom Kippur, no less). "Even if someone had a cigarette three days ago, I can tell," Mungara says, and it dawns on me that although I think his room smells funny, all minty male sports cream, he probably thinks I smell worse—and he's right.

One more reason the Kenyan marathon runners have been so successful is that they egg each other on. As each guy breaks a new record, they lower the ceiling on possibilities. It's like wanting to become a rapper and being from Brooklyn. You grow up seeing it done. "The great thing about Kenya is that it's not just one or two guys you can run with that are fast, there's lots of them," says Reid Coolsaet, who goes to Kenya to train for a month after Christmas every year. "It's so different out there—no distractions. Everyone runs," he says. "It's part of the culture, so getting up early, eating well, avoiding alcohol and fast food, spending lots of time running, and then recovering from the run isn't seen as crazy—it's what everyone does." Hang around with a lot of runners and you're apt to run more. Run with a group and it's not as hard getting out of the house. That's how my friends Betty Lee and Lesley Taylor got to the marathon.

In Ottawa, I ran with Silas Sang and Hosea Rotich, two elite Kenyan marathoners, and Rotich told me I run like a rhinoceros, as I watched him prance around on his midfoot like he was skipping across hot coals. (I also heard the story of how Rotich started running. He was working as a forest ranger and spotted Simon Wangai, one of Kenya's top distance guys, chopping down trees. Rotich, who was wearing a tool belt and work boots, took off after him. Wangai was impressed, and encouraged Rotich to quit forestry and run marathons.) Harvard's Daniel Lieberman and Irene Davis would approve of Rotich's form: this is the technique of the caveman, and minimalist sneakers encourage you to land this way, on the midfoot, on the balls of your feet.

I'm not saying you should change your foot strike two weeks away from your race. Reid Coolsaet lands on his heels, and he's done all right. So does Kenneth Mungara, and he's done even better. I run like a hippopotamus and I can still tough out a marathon. But that's something to think about on your next run. How are you landing? Try not to shake the branches from the trees.

Also, Mungara, Sang, Rotich, Korir—these guys are always smiling. For them, races are real pressure: they actually do run to win. And when I meet them, it's usually after a long flight and they may not understand exactly what I'm saying. (Most of my friends don't, and some of us have known each other since we went to the same high school together.) Still, they let me ask personal questions and make dumb observations while we watch ads on TV. They usually take me out on a run. Once I had a bug in my eye on a run with Nzinga, and he used a blade of grass to get it out. I don't think I could do that for Esme. Keep things natural and keep things mellow. Live like a Kenyan. We run better when we're calm.

Here's one last thing I've learned about determination from African runners. Koren Yal is one of six siblings raised on her parents' farm in Ethiopia, and after she won a marathon in Mumbai with a prize of $36,000, I asked her why Ethiopians and Kenyans seem to be such good long-distance racers. "Running is my job," says Yal, who grew up in awe of Derartu Tulu, Ethiopia's star female runner, who won the 2009 New York City Marathon. I tell her that the average household income of the New York Marathon participant is over $100,000 and ask her if that disparity might work in her favor. After all, when Geoffrey Mutai finished first at the New York City Marathon in 2011 and then won the World Marathon Majors—that is, he accumulated the most points from his finishes at the six biggest marathons around the world (Boston, London, Berlin, Chicago, New York, and Tokyo)—collecting $500,000, he didn't elevate his standard of living. He still slept on the floor of his training camp, along with fifteen other men. "To run, you need a big motivation," says Yal. "Money in your pocket is motivation."

Think about your motivation and adjust your goals accordingly. Malcolm Gladwell has written about running himself nearly unconscious while racing as a teenager, after which, he decided he never wanted to feel that way again. We have limits about what we want to endure. That's fine. Just remember those limits when you set your goals.

"We control our own fate," says Kenneth Mungara, and it's hard not to listen—on race day, he wins the Toronto Marathon once again.

THE SOUNDTRACK: Michael Bublé
Michael Bublé has soft pink skin, and he sits on a love seat in the Ritz-Carlton hotel as if it were the most natural place for him in the world. He's recently married an Argentine supermodel, but when we meet Bublé is in town to promote his Christmas album, which will become one of the best-selling discs of the year. As we chat, he's complaining about the toll running takes on his knees: "I just can't do it outside anymore—it's hell on my joints," he says. I try to convince him that maybe he's just wearing the wrong shoes or else falling for the anti-running hype. He refuses to budge: "I love running," he says, "but for me it has to be on the treadmill."

Listen to Michael Bublé's love songs. If he hosts the Junos again, tune in. But I think you can discount his advice about running. The Argentine supermodel didn't marry him because of how fast he finished his 10K.

"Gold Digger," Kanye West: "I've never met Kanye West, but I love him and I love this song. It's got a great beat and, of course, you can't knock the concept. It's pretty funny… something to think about while you run."

"All Over the World," Electric Light Orchestra: "It reminds me of being in gym class in Grade 4."

"Footloose," Kenny Loggins: "Again—gym class. Do you know anyone who doesn't love this song?"

13

RACE TWO, RUNNING BEATEN: TORONTO

ROUNDING THE CORNER at Mile 19 of the Toronto Marathon, I run into a gale-force wind. I know it's coming—my adversaries have been gossiping about it the entire race. But nothing can prepare you for the forces of nature—especially when you're at your most tired, feeling your most beaten down.

I run the marathon on October 16, and it's the first time I'm not really sure if I'll finish. The race gets underway as most do: the starting line's crowded and people fight to make space. I'm in my lucky outfit—gray shorts with built-in black underwear and a little pocket for race gels; and a nice lightweight white shirt with stains in the underarms that won't wash away. I'm wearing neutral, lightweight—not minimalist—sneakers and competing against other reporters in the media challenge division, which I won last year. The winner gets $1,000 for their favorite charity, and mine is Julie's dad's church. Esme's with Julie's sister, and Julie's with her parents (and their congregation) somewhere around 39K (24 miles).

The morning is dark—cold and somber. And by the time I reach 5K (3 miles), I'm well out in front of my 3:10 pacer. It's a mistake I make almost every race, but today I'm gunning for a Boston-qualifying time and it's hard to keep my nerves under wraps. I always feel amazing when a race begins, adrenaline hitting me like a shot of cocaine. I know it won't last. How can it with thirty-seven more kilometers to go? But, nevertheless, here I am, blazing. Feeling like this is the marathon in which I will break all my records. At 5K, that's about the stupidest thought in the world.

There are lots of spectators, and I enjoy hot-dogging. It's a thrill giving them high-fives and smiles all the way through the run's first half. I fight against the wind for the first 10K (6 miles), then get pushed by the wind at my back until 32K (20 miles). Ten kilometers into my run, I'm thinking about coming in under three hours. I slept well the evening before the race, which I never do, and even though my training wasn't terrific, I feel confident. Last month, I ran a strong half, and who's to say how fast I can run this morning? I see my friend with his boy on his shoulders, and I swoop in and give the kid five.

There's a group of guys from Halifax trying to finish at 3:05, and I run with them for a while, until we make our first loop at 12K (7 miles). Breezy conversation makes the kilometers disappear... At this point, I can see the elites Kenneth Mungara, Reid Coolsaet, and my friend Matt Loiselle who have already made their turn. I call out their names, but none of them looks in my direction. Mungara might drink tea slowly and watch cop shows, but he transforms when it's time to race. I don't think he'd turn his head to watch Lady Gaga perform.

I'm still running well out in front of my pacer at 15K (9.3 miles) and feeling like I can run a three-hour marathon. I run my quickest 5K on the straightaway, with the wind at my back, to the halfway point—17 to 22 (10 to 13 miles)—and I'm marveling at how good I feel. I know the 25K (15-mile) mark's going to be a killer. I'm running down Cherry Street across this horrible metal water bridge, and it's desolate and shot with wind, and when I get to the 25K mark, things start to change. The run starts to feel long.

How does it happen? One step I'm Iron Man, and the next step I'm screwed. Some people say the marathon doesn't even start until 30K (18 miles). On this day, it began for me at twenty-six.

A HALF-MARATHON is a civil distance to compete in. The full marathon is pain. I take my first gooey energy gel just past the roundabout, on Cherry, and make it through the halfway point. Now, for the first time in this race, I have to remind myself to relax. I focus on keeping my knees up, on swinging my arms, on looking forward, and on breathing—on trying to stay calm.

At the beginning, the run didn't require any effort. It felt like an invisible river was just pulling me along. But now I'm caught in the struggle, going against the tide, and I'm calculating and recalculating how far I have left to go. The guys from Halifax pull away from me, and though I'm scared to look back, I sense the 3:10 pacer's approaching like the wave of guilt that hits when I first wake up after a very long night. It sucks knowing that I'm getting slower, that I'm tired and hurting, because I need to reach 32K before the hard part of the race begins.

I've never fallen during a marathon. I've never had to walk, and I've never pulled over to either throw up or use the john. I haven't hit the Wall, haven't run out of glycogen, haven't stepped on a rock or worn the wrong thing—I've just been running an awfully long distance in an awfully short time, and I feel like I want to find a nice warm place to curl up and hide.

Usually I'm smiling and trying to engage the spectators, throwing my little cups of Gatorade in the trash. But that last straightaway in the wind, at 32K, is a chamber of horrors. It requires everything, and everything I have isn't enough. I can't reach down like in some motivational running advertisement, and when I pop my second energy gel it doesn't do a damned thing. Now the spectators are annoying. It's like I'm jogging through quicksand and every kilometer finds me leaking just a little more time... 35... 36... 37... The race seems to be taking an eternity. I push forward and reach the Greek cheering station, where I put on half of a brave face. I'm wobbling more than running. And though I don't have any cramps or specific pains or injuries, I just feel an overall heaviness. Like I'm running with Esme's crib on my back.

At the half-marathon, I was passing people left and right toward the finish line. Picking people off like a fighter plane. This time, there's nothing in the tank, and even when I reach the 41K (25-mile) mark, when I can smell the finish line and the spectators are saying, "You're almost there," and "Looking good, keep going," I can't dig any farther. My hips feel like they're made of porcelain, and each step threatens to bring the whole china cabinet that's become my body crashing down. When did my sneakers become concrete slabs?

Still, I keep pushing—my body shivering, my skin becoming evermore greenish-yellow, my stomach burning—and remain vertical across the finish line, before I collapse into a volunteer's tinfoil jacket. I crossed the finish line setting my own personal record, 3:08:40—enough to earn my berth to Boston—but I'm freezing and it's all I can do to stumble into the first available port-a-potty and release a stream of diarrhea. I shake continually, despite the cheap aluminum heat blanket. Finally I meet up with Julie and her parents, and I feel like an old bag of bones left out on the street, waiting to be picked up in a Toronto green bin as compost. When I try to put on my sweatpants, my right calf muscle seizes up and I can't move my leg. Out of nowhere, a guy with baby dreadlocks steps forward and administers a massage. When I can move again, I rush off once more to the bathroom. I eat a banana and drink water and Gatorade.

On the ride home, fighting traffic, we hear about the twenty-seven-year-old who died during the race. I get home, take a bath and two Advil, and eat two slices of pizza, four skewers of souvlaki and potato salad, and then order Chinese.

I'm glad Mungara won his third straight marathon in Toronto. And it's amazing that Coolsaet and Eric Gillis qualified for the Olympic Games. Hats off to all 22,000 runners who competed. Hats off to you on reaching 10K.

God knows it isn't easy—at least it wasn't for me.

THREE

LOVE THE PAIN

CONQUERING THE HALF-MARATHON

"On the road again/just can't wait
to get on the road again."

WILLIE NELSON, a runner, probably around 800 million
times since writing his Grammy Award-winning hit in 1980
(see his music selections, page 159)

BUILDING
YOUR NETWORK

THE TRAINING: Work Out Like an Adult (Based on Distance, not Time)

WEEK 27: Three times this week, run 7K (4.3 miles), being consistent and building your base. Sign up for your half and invest in a pedometer that keeps track of your pace and total distance per run. Since we all run at different speeds, from now on the workouts will be based on distance, not time. Walk proudly, as ever, where you have to.

WEEK 28: Run 7K twice this week and try to hit 9K (5.6 miles) on your third run.

WEEK 29: Run three times this week: a 7K run, a second 7K run (or hills or speed work), and a long run of 10K (6.2 miles).

THE SOUNDTRACK: Slash

THE FINISH LINE: The half, now just about 13 weeks away.

IF YOU'VE been running for six months and have completed two races, congratulations. If you've done that, you don't need to hear anything from me—and yet, *mazel tov*, I hope your legs are sore but you're walking tall. What you've finished is an accomplishment, and by getting this far your ultimate goal is now just six months away. Halfway to the finish line, already successful, your most exhilarating races are still to come.

Sign up for your half-marathon now so that you can establish a timeframe for reaching your marathon, the big enchilada. It's in your grasp. Your training in this section will take place over three months, and if you can go out three times this week for 7K (4.3 miles), you can be ready for 21K (13.1 miles) in thirteen weeks. Running 7K three times this week will make you strong enough to run 10K (6.2 miles) once next week. Each step forward is a building block, and we're just adding little distances one foot after the other and week after week. Next week, hit 7K twice and then run 9K (5.6 miles). After that, Week 29 for those still following along from the beginning, run 7K again, and then once more, or else try speed work or hills, and then tough out a long run of 10K.

Once you can run 17K (10.5 miles), the thinking goes that you can run 21.09K (13.1 miles), so our long run this section will top out at 19K (11.8 miles), just to be safe. By running 7K a few times this week, you're building to within striking distance of that magic seventeen goal. You can do this. It's just small incremental steps like it has been. However, there's a pretty big difference between 10K and the half-marathon. Distance, sure, but mental stamina too. It tests your level of commitment, your guts, your drive. The training's about to get tougher, so now's a good time to run with a friend.

"LOSERS!" SHOUTS a man at the Black Bull, a bar with a huge outside patio on Queen Street West in Toronto, the fat center of the city's booming west side. I'm running around with about forty people and the sun hasn't set yet, and not a single member of the Longboat Roadrunners seems to hear what the man's said. I admit we look somewhat peculiar—there's a guy nearing seventy in a singlet with great patches of white hair sprouting like dandelions all over his shoulders, and a woman in heavy makeup who looks like she might be on the run from the cops.

Our group hangs a left on Blue Jays Way and, as a posse, like a herd of ostrich, we pass the baseball fans with their oversized fingers and gloves on their way to the stadium to see the Jays. People stare, but the men and women of Longboat just keep running until we hit the waterfront, where the runners break off into subgroups. Some people are running fast and short distances; others, like the guy with long hair who ran a 100-mile race this past Sunday—today's Wednesday— are doing a slow 16K (10 miles). I hang with these guys and meet Bert de Vries, now sixty-five and the founder of the club.

"We started because of beer," says de Vries, who used to be a member of the University of Toronto's track club but formed a rival band when the team—which also consisted of pole vaulters, shotputters, and the men and women who throw discus and javelins—wouldn't spring for a few cases of suds for the distance runners bussing out to Ottawa for a meet. "We were going to start something new that would be egalitarian— about teamwork—and nurture distance runners who might want a beer every now and again," says de Vries, retired from teaching high school Latin. "I knew we needed something different. It would be as much a social as a running thing."

It's easier to do something hard with other people. The Longboat Roadrunners encourage each other, share information, lend support and coaching advice, and have created a community that its members respect. You don't skip a run, because that's not what the club's about. There's pride there. Remember, it's one thing to train for 10K in isolation. But it helps to have someone by your side to complete the half-marathon.

Early on, my running buddy, Ben, and I decided we'd run to work together on Tuesday and Thursday mornings, 20K (12.8 miles), through whatever. If it's raining, we run. If our wives are nine months pregnant, we run. If we've had seven gin and tonics the night before, we know we're running. Neither of us calls in a sick day, and neither of us cancels a run. We didn't say it, but this is the contract we signed, and you have to. Once you start making allowances, momentum dissolves and, out of nowhere, that 20K becomes something you used to do, for a while. Like that friend you meant to call or that book you were so excited to read, this is the way shoes remain in the closet.

SO HOW do you find someone to run with? The easiest thing is to sign up for a clinic, run for a charity, or join a run club. Since so many more people are running, many organizations offer help. In the U.S., try runningintheusa.com; in England, runengland.org; in Canada, check out runningroom.com; and in Hong Kong, because who knows, see hkrunners.com. If your tastes lean toward the lighthearted, investigate the Hash House Harriers (gotothehash.net), an international organization started in 1938 in Malaysia that bills itself as a "drinking club with a running problem." There are also running groups operating out of the YMCA, community centers, shops like Lululemon and Nike and, in Canada, MEC. Meanwhile, charity groups are transforming the sport. In 2012, running and walking events raised more than $1.68 billion. Want motivation? Try running for somebody else. In Ottawa, there's even a run club for the blind, and at ChristianRunners.org, you can find faith-based running groups in five American cities, Toronto, and the Dominican Republic.

You may not be much of a joiner. Christie Blatchford, the Canadian journalist, prides herself on being an iconoclast. "I typically hate most people and particularly hate women, but when I decided to do the marathon, I knew I needed some help," says Blatchford, who joined a running club in 2005 to train for a marathon and then, two years later, separated from the pack and formed her own splinter cell, picking and choosing her members. Blatchford writes about the most gruesome crimes in Canada, and she followed the troops through two tours in Afghanistan, but even she finds it hard to drag herself out alone at 5:30 a.m. in cold, wet November weather to run 15K before work.

"It's not like I was looking to make friends or improve my social life—though, in the end, I did both of those things— I just needed a boost from someone to help me drag my ass out there," Blatchford says. The members of her group pride themselves on never missing a session, and I join them one morning while the moon's still out. They come for the camaraderie. The running's almost something they receive on the side. "Guys can play sports and develop friendships, but for women, especially in the middle of your life, developing real intimacy is hard," one of Blatchford's friends tells me as we kibitz our way through a cold early morning jog.

For five consecutive years (2006–2010), Running USA reports, the number of half-marathon finishers in North America has grown annually by 10 percent. In 2012, the number of finishers increased by 14.9 percent. Since 2000, the number of half-marathon finishers has nearly tripled (it's gone up 284 percent), and in 2012, 60 percent of half-marathon finishers were women. (This is why, in the past decade, the half-marathon has become North America's fastest-growing distance to race.) Five kilometers is still the most popular event, but the half attracts more runners than the 10K. That means you can do this. Why else would people be coming out for it in droves?

More numbers: the average half-marathon female finisher is 35.3 years old and takes an average time of almost two hours and twenty minutes to complete her race. The average male finisher is 38.2 and takes just about an even two hours to finish, more time than you can knock off by running around your block alone once or twice a few times. Because the novelty of running will wear off and the honeymoon will fade, it's going to be beneficial to find more than just me and this book for encouragement.

"We're social beings, we like to connect with people, and it doesn't hurt to use a group to pace ourselves, push ourselves, and provide positive peer pressure not to skip a run," says Jeff Brown, assistant clinical professor of psychiatry at Harvard Medical School and the official psychologist of the Boston Marathon. (And how's that for crazy? Even before the bombing, the marathon attracted so many people it had its own shrink.)

When asked why people might like to run in a group, Brown refers to the animal kingdom: "Dare I say that wild animals run in packs when they have a goal of hunting things down, and perhaps we have a similar goal, in that we're hunting down the end of a race?" He adds that clusters of runners form during the half-marathon and that complete strangers end up running together, not only in the middle or the back of the group but also among the group's leaders.

How is it that 25,000 people can begin a race together across 21K and the finishers all cross the line in great clumps separated only by seconds? "There's an affiliation we have with others in a similar situation, with similar goals, especially with noncompetitive, middle-of-the-pack runners. When the competition's been eliminated, we share a combined purpose—the idea is to work together," Brown tells me, adding that there's a guardian angel phenomenon that occurs during races, in which complete strangers become coach, confidant, mother, and best friend. "Time after time we hear about races where runners will meet someone, someone whom at the start of the race they didn't know, who ends up helping them through—or even saving them, if you'd prefer—those tough last four miles. Whatever it is that bonds people—almost like with soldiers in a war zone—occurs when we run the marathon or the half."

The Road Runners Club of America was formed in 1958 in New York with ten people. It currently has more than a thousand chapters and 200,000 members across the country. Traditionally, shoe shops have been the natural incubator for running groups, and when Nike was known as Blue Ribbon Sports in Eugene, Oregon, runners would converge and train together at the shop.

John Stanton, founder of Canada's Running Room chain says, "I started the first clinic right when I opened the first store. I think people realized they could go from couch potato to athlete if they just had a little support." He now estimates that almost 70 percent of his customers enroll in one of the Learn to Run clinics at his 140 stores across Canada and the U.S. To date, he's had 800,000 people take his classes—about thirty couples meet this way every year—and for his work helping to make people more active, he's been awarded the Order of Canada.

"A lot of us have enough stress in our workplace and want running to be fun, to add to our quality of life, not take away from it, and the running groups have added a social aspect that's done just that," says Stanton, a former pack-a-day smoker. Before opening the Running Room, he got his start in Edmonton's grocery store business, and he says the clinics, which meet twice a week and train runners from the 5K to the marathon, were inspired by in-store demonstrations he'd done to sell everything from stainless steel cookware to perogies filled with potatoes and cheese. In the grocery business, "we always called it 'show and sell.' If you show customers the benefits of a product, that helps the sell," says Stanton, who used to teach every clinic at the Edmonton Running Room store. When he opened his second store in Calgary, Stanton drove from his home in Edmonton every Saturday morning to teach class. Eventually, to turn his sales force into trainers, Stanton began to write books. Today, his signature 10-and-1 training formula—you walk one minute after every ten minutes of running, all the way to the marathon—is followed all over the country.

"Running groups provide structure and positive peer pressure; we're committed not only to ourselves but to a group," Stanton says. "It's like when you're a kid and you join a soccer team—running becomes playful as opposed to something arduous. And it's not only fun, but it helps you achieve your goals."

I could probably run without Ben but I don't want to. Some weeks, I talk to him more than anyone other than my wife. You don't need an instructor to reach the half-marathon. You can follow this book and make it all the way to 42.2K. But the journey will require less resolve if you're not gutting out each mile all by yourself. Recruit a partner. Enlist a co-worker. Run with a friend.

"IF YOU TRAIN with friends, you'll be more motivated," says Josphat Nzinga, who grew up in the sticks of Kenya but moved to Nyahururu, where the country's best distance runners work together informally twice a day. He says that anyone's welcome to the free run club, which is held without coaches or sponsors. In 1993, Cosmas Ndeti, Nzinga's uncle, won the Boston Marathon. When he returned home, he went right back to running with his friends—only he was able to distribute contacts and shoes.

"People who run well and have money help other people who are trying to make a life far from their village," Nzinga tells me, as we sit in Julie's mom's car outside his building after a run. "When I got to Nyahururu, I moved from one house to another. Since I was running in the morning and afternoon, I didn't have time to look for work and didn't have any food." Eventually he was hired by Patrick Makau as a masseur and driver. Makau ran 2011's Berlin Marathon in 2:03:38, the fastest marathon finish of all time. However, more important than breaking the world record was the cash prize he earned for his victory: 40,000 euros. With that money, he hired his friend. "If I'm at the training camp and don't have money, I have to talk to Makau. This morning we finished two hours of training, but in my home right now I don't have anything to eat. If he has anything, he'll help me—that's the way it always has been."

Nzinga's uncle was part of this system, and so was Sammy Wanjiru, the youngest marathon gold medal winner in seventy-six years. In Kenya, the runners motivate each other and train together, constantly pushing the pace and also swapping information: Which marathon offers the biggest prizes? What shoe company is looking for athletes? How do the Americans train? This is what you want to replicate in your own group. Everyone helps each other. Everyone is responsible to the team. Everyone shows up ready to work. And, when you need a little extra motivation, you can count on your friends. They're literally walking in your same shoes.

"Everyone's in charge and we give responsibilities to everyone. At the end of the year, everyone's running better," Nzinga says. "If you fool around, people are going to dismiss you, but if you work hard, you benefit from running with the group."

From your running group, look for consistency. You want people you can depend on—they don't have to be fast, but they do have to show up on time. It helps if someone in the group has completed the distance you're training for, and it's good when at least two or three members go at roughly the same speed. I like running with people faster than me, but twice I've had to quit running with fast friends because they just lived too far away. The group's got to be convenient and the meeting times have to work with your schedule. Otherwise, it'll be impossible to sustain.

When hiring a running coach (kaplan.ben@gmail.com), make certain it's someone who understands kinesiology and ask your doctor about the advice before signing a check. A coach should educate and inspire, push you beyond what you're capable of on your own, and pace you while you train. If your club, coach, trainer, or buddy doesn't make you love running, drop 'em. Being miserable you can do on your own.

For Christie Blatchford, a running group took her well beyond the marathon. In the seven years that her gang has been training, they've skipped only one run. That day Blatchford was working on her book and fighting through writer's block, and instead of running, her pals sat with her around a kitchen table and helped shape her material into an outline that would lead to a Governor General's Award. The book, *Fifteen Days*, is dedicated to the soldiers. It's also dedicated to her running club.

"Running with a group can push you beyond your capacity, or even what you think your capacity is," says Bert de Vries over a beer with his Longboat Roadrunners after we finish our Wednesday night run. "You build up your confidence—if they can do it, I can too." As I'm leaving to go home, some of the Longboats head out for a nightcap at a bar in the area. We're not far from the Black Bull, and this gets me thinking: members of the Longboat Roadrunners may find themselves sitting next to the guy who called us losers. The only difference between him and us is this: we can all run a marathon.

THE SOUNDTRACK: Slash

My interview with Slash has been my most-read story of all the people in this book, including Justin Bieber and Katy Perry. The guy is just bad, and he has actual firsthand experience with Axl, music's biggest psycho since Tupac Shakur.

I was nervous about meeting him, and it was not easy asking him questions about running, especially after being instructed not to ask him any questions about Axl and then asking him those questions one after the other as his publicist cringed. Slash is a big dude, even without the top hat, and he doesn't suffer fools, but whatever. He may not have loved our interview, but check out the circumstances surrounding how he wrote "Sweet Child O' Mine."

"We were living in this house with no furniture, and I was sitting on the floor, playing my guitar and working on this riff. It was late afternoon," says Slash. "Izzy had his guitar and he played some chords behind it. Duff was there, and Axl was upstairs, and I guess he overheard it; it was really a passing thing." The next day, Guns N' Roses went into rehearsal. "Axl said, 'Play that thing you guys were working on yesterday.' I guess it inspired him to write some lyrics, and 'Sweet Child O' Mine' started to blossom."

So Axl really is special?

"'Genius' is a good word."

This is his spiel about running: "I hate running. I run. But I hate running and I hate the iPod; I just watch TV," he said. "I do it and get it over with. I hate exercise."

If you weren't watching television, and not on an iPod, what would you listen to?

"Anything hard-driving—Metallica, Slayer, Megadeth. *Reign in Blood* is my favorite Slayer record, but they've got a lot of good records. *Garage Days Revisited* by Metallica, or else *Master of Puppets*. And for Megadeth, let's say *Peace Sells... But Who's Buying?*, which is one of their biggest records but also my favorite. And if you want to go run up a mountain, listen to Lamb of God or Mastodon. That's heavy stuff."

15

THE CROSS-TRAINING APPEAL

THE TRAINING: Run Farther, Run Less

WEEK 30: Try an 8K (5-mile) run, walking if you have to, and 30 minutes on a rowing machine (or else 30 minutes cycling or swimming), and a 12K (7.4-mile) long run.

WEEK 31: Get serious, one 8K run, 40 minutes on a bike, and a long run of 13K (8.1 miles).

THE SOUNDTRACK: Brian Wilson

THE FINISH LINE: A half-marathon, now just about 10 weeks away.

NEARLY ALL of the experts agree that you can reduce the risk of a running injury by simply running less. It makes sense; if you cook less, you're less likely to get burned by the stove. That said, about two months away from the half-marathon is no time to slow down. This is a conundrum. Increase your volume, and you increase the likelihood of something bad happening. But you need to increase your volume to run greater distances. Or do you? Many top athletes and kinesiology experts are becoming more and more receptive to the idea of quality, not just quantity, of training. In the '70s, marathoners ran like a Rockette's stocking, clocking as many as 320 kilometers (200 miles) a week. Today, an increasing number of top distance runners are decreasing their miles while increasing their supplemental workouts. Cross-training—augmenting your running with something like swimming, cycling, and arm exercises with weights—will help you better enjoy your half-marathon.

"If you do nothing but train for one specific thing, eventually that thing is going to have some negative consequences," says Dr. Jonathan Chang, orthopedic surgeon and professor of medicine at the University of Southern California. A distance runner nearly fast enough to qualify for the Olympics, Chang is a member of the American College of Sports Medicine and says too often he sees injured runners coming by his clinic with plantar fasciitis (inflamed feet), shin splints (stressed muscles around the tibia), and knee pain (knee pain). He's constantly advising runners to swim, ride a bike, use an elliptical machine, or circuit-train with light weights. (Runners don't want bulky muscles; bulky anything, even muscle mass, hinders speed.)

"In order to get good at something it takes practice, but you can take things too far," Chang tells me. "Hence, cross-train."

Chang's favorite exercise for runners is using the rowing machine, which works out the arms, shoulders, back, quadriceps, and core (your upper and lower abdominals), and encourages your upper and lower body to work in unison while avoiding the loading stress of a run. It's also a great way to burn calories. Since we're building up to a 13K (8.1-mile) long run next week, augment one run with a thirty-minute session on a rowing machine. Don't worry if 13K feels difficult; it's far. And please walk for a minute or two every ten minutes rather than quit. Our goal, really, to ace the half-marathon is 17K (10.5 miles) in practice, so thirteen is a significant accomplishment. Hit thirteen, and you're gold. You're still running twice this week, but varying the exercise will provide some relief to your joints while working on your cardiovascular system and building strength. It's a good plan.

Next week, as you continue to lengthen your long run, use the rowing machine again for about thirty minutes or, if one isn't available, cycle or swim. Both exercises can be swapped with a run without short-changing your overall conditioning, and, if you normally run for, say, forty-five minutes, spend that same amount of time on a bike or in the pool.

"I've run through nine years, ten marathons, and three kids, and I'm about an hour faster now than when I started," says Krista DuChene, who began swimming in 2004 when she was injured just before the Boston Marathon and was hoping to finish around 3:28. Today, DuChene trains between ten and sixteen hours a week and spends three of those days in the pool, both pool running and swimming laps. Pool running looks so awkward that it makes running up and down your neighbor's hill look suave, but if you mimic your running form in the pool's deep end and keep your heart and stride rate consistent with that of a run (130 to 180 strides per minute), you'll exercise the same muscle groups with zero impact. Try sprinting for one minute after every ten minutes of pool jogging and do that for thirty minutes once a week. Do that, and you might become like Krista DuChene, who ran the 2012 Rotterdam Marathon in 2:32, one of the top-ten fastest marathon finishes of all time by a Canadian woman. (Again, she's a mother of three.)

"I'd think everyone could benefit from that type of workout. It's made me a better athlete, and I can feel the extra strength in my core when I run," she says. "The reason I started swimming is that was the only thing I was allowed to do while injured—just to keep my sanity when all I wanted to do was run—but it's a good life lesson and I've stuck with swimming ever since. It helps prevent the excess stress on your body."

Swimming is a good exercise for runners because it works the heart, lungs, arms, shoulders, legs, and core, and cycling is terrific because, in addition to the cardiovascular workout, when you cycle up a hill, standing on the pedals as you climb, it mimics the exact motion as when you jog. If you're circuit-training, a good runner's workout would include pull-ups, bench presses, and squats, exercises that train movement muscles, according to Jason Fitzgerald's book *101 Simple Ways to Be a Better Runner*.

Ten weeks to the half-marathon, twenty-three weeks to the marathon, hopefully you're beginning to see this stuff as building blocks for the long haul. No one thing makes you fit. It's a cumulative effort. So keep documenting your training and adding distance, with respectful caution, as you decide which marathon you might choose to run. Almost every city has one, from Beirut to Belfast, and I'm sure there's a great race where you live. Where do you want to end up when you finish?

"When you don't want to run another second, it can be easy to get in the pool or on the bike, which helps with recovery and is a good way to build different muscles," says John Honerkamp, who writes the official online training program of the New York City Marathon and recommends that everybody, but especially new runners or athletes carrying a few extra pounds, try cross-country skiing, spin class, Zumba, pole dancing, or something like active yoga along with their runs. "You need long runs to get to the marathon, that's no question, but cross-training will help you to run more. It's about not killing yourself in the beginning but strengthening everything, including your mind."

So much of what I like about running is the metaphor, and all that has to do with perseverance and the long haul. I've started bringing Esme to baby music class, and when we took her to New York, it was one of the happiest moments of my life. There were all sorts of highs, including a drink with Aunt Linda, but nothing could touch seeing my parents as grandparents for the first time. My mom wanted to do nothing other than hold baby Esme, even when the band played Motown. And my father—I'll never forget this—watched me bring Esme down a long, winding flight of stairs after a feeding, holding onto her like she was a coat and I was freezing, and when I got to the bottom, knocking away a bead of sweat, my dad said, "You know, I don't think I could've done that. You and Julie are doing a great job."

I was not doing a great job when I started. I couldn't collapse the stroller. I left flecks of milk in the bottles when I washed them. I tried to install the car seat, and when Julie finally took it to the firehall to get some help, the guys all gathered around to see the mess that I'd made. But you can't quit. It takes effort to improve, of course, but mostly practice. And dogged determination and fire and refusing to give up, give in. You just have to make the decision that this is something you're going to do, and then do it, despite whatever, and if you diversify your practice, you can practice for longer, practice until you get good—and achieve mastery. Cross-training, in essence, is a runner's survival tool. You need to keep your workouts fresh.

"Whenever I try and function like a robot, it never works. So much comes down to happiness and stress levels, even in my sporting life," says Sarah Groff, the American triathlete who finished fourth at the London Olympic Games. Groff's interesting because, after earning her career's best finish in 2012, she parted ways with her coach and traded in her performance training in Australia to move to New Hampshire with her boyfriend, Ben. Sarah knows all about cross-training: she bikes, swims, and runs for something like twenty-five hours a week. And she says she'd never be able to be completely monogamous to any one discipline. The rewards she reaps from having multiple sporting partners are too rich. "Doing a single sport can feel tedious, like work, but by doing different workouts, it keeps it fun and exciting," she says. "Besides, I could never be cool with just running. Triathletes look much better in a bikini."

THE SOUNDTRACK: Brian Wilson

The Beach Boys' Brian Wilson is probably the most brilliant and most screwed-up individual you'll meet in this book. Forget about all of his own tunes, the guy inspired The Beatles to write *Sgt. Pepper*. I could go on and on about him. I remember when my parents took my sister and me to see him every summer at Merriweather Post Pavilion during his band's "Kokomo" days, and next to Paul Simon and Bob Dylan, he's done as much as anybody to influence pop music's sound.

"I exercise every day," he says, when we speak on the phone before his show in Toronto. Wilson was in Los Angeles on his way to the studio, and he wasn't sure exactly what he would be recording, but it turned out to be a track for the brilliant *Listen to Me: Buddy Holly* tribute album. "I like walking around the park. It keeps your mind healthy and keeps your brain clear. I like taking walks," Wilson said, and the exercise seemed to pay dividends. After he played in Toronto, the reunited Beach Boys performed at the Grammys and then released *That's Why God Made the Radio*, which pretty much got panned, but I kind of like it anyway.

Interviewing Wilson's a bit like interviewing a lamppost, but I was able to get him to recommend two running songs.

"'Let It Be' by The Beatles and 'Be My Baby' by the Ronettes and Phil Spector," he said. "These are the songs that make me the happiest. They'd be good for a run."

DURING AN interview with David Felton for *Rolling Stone* on November 4, 1976, Brian Wilson explained why he runs.

The world is messed up. How do you deal with it?
BRIAN: The way I deal with it is I go jogging in the morning. I goddamn get out of bed and I jog, and I make sure I stay in shape. That's how I do it. And so far the only way I've been keeping from drugs is with those bodyguards, and the only way I've been going jogging is those bodyguards have been taking me jogging.
So in one sense you're not yet fully committed to the idea.
BRIAN: It's just that once you've had a taste of drugs, you like 'em and you want 'em. Do you take drugs yourself?
Yeah, I experiment.
BRIAN: Do ya? Do ya snort?
See, now I guess you gotta get to the point in the program where you're not going to ask me questions like that.
BRIAN: That's right. You just saw my weakness coming out. Which I don't understand. I just do it anyway. I used to drink my head off too, that's another thing. They've been keeping me from drinkin', taking pills, and taking coke. And I'm jogging every morning.

This excerpt appears courtesy of David Felton. Thanks, David. Check out the complete story online: www.rollingstone.com/music/news/the-healing-of-brother-brian-the-rolling-stone-interview-with-the-beach-boys-19761104

16

THE
RUNNER'S CODE

THE TRAINING: Going Hard

WEEK 32: Run 3 times: an 8K (5 miles), an 8K that includes four 20-second fartleks, and a long run of 14K (8.7 miles).

WEEK 33: Here, incorporate your cross-training: run 8K, then try 35 minutes of rowing (or swimming or biking), and finish the week with an 11K (6.8-mile) long run.

WEEK 34: The long run is the thing. Try 8K twice, slow and easy, then rest up for a long run of 16K (10 miles).

THE SOUNDTRACK: Metric

THE FINISH LINE: The half, now just about 7 weeks away.

WITHIN TWO months of your half-marathon, in addition to your 8K (5-mile) easy workout and the 8K you're running with four twenty-second bursts of speed—you're doing that, right?—the long run tops out at 16K (10 miles), damn near close to seventeen, our magic number. You're pushing things now and the training is tough, so next week be sure that you cross-train. Choose swimming or cycling to augment your runs—or rowing, if possible, because that's the best overall workout. Explore the farthest reaches of your talent—if something's going to happen, if you're going to push too hard and/ or run out of steam, better it happen in practice than in the half-marathon itself. How will you respond to the pain?

This week, try 14K (8.7 miles) on your long run, and do 8K twice, with a series of fartleks, say four of them for twenty seconds, when you feel like the universe isn't meting out the rewards you deserve. The following week, drop your long run down to 11K (6.8 miles) and work in some cross-training, whether it's the rowing machine, the pool, or the bike. Finally, in your thirty-fourth week of training, take two 8K runs slowly and rest up for your long run. Here, break all your records and run 16K, packing water and bus fare. Take it slowly. Walk when you need to, but attempt to complete the whole route, and pretend it's the race. Don't let the distance take you by surprise on game day.

EVERY TUESDAY and Thursday, when Ben and I run in to work, we cut through the city for 5K and then go north along the Don Valley ravine for another 12K before again hitting the street. Twice, beside the brook, I've seen deer, and we've also seen rabbits and hedgehogs, a fox, and a snake. One time, a red-winged blackbird pecked at my bald spot, and after I shooed it away and ran on, it swooped in after me again. I was in such a bad mood that morning, I'm sure it was going after my vibes.

The path's never crowded, but it is frequently used by bikers, dog walkers, even a class of runners—a group of older women tethered together. I've never been able to figure out if it's because one of the groups of two includes a blind runner.

Or maybe it's to ensure someone will be there if one of them falls. I keep meaning to ask.

One morning, we noticed a couple of signs. The first one was written in blue ink and red magic marker on a piece of white paper, placed inside a sealed plastic bag, and duct-taped to a post. It read: "Found: Garmin. Saturday, June 16" with a phone number. I thought that was cool. Someone found a watch, and instead of pocketing it, took the trouble to go home, make a sign, return to the path, and post it. Awesome.

The story gets better. Beneath that sign was another one, written a little more crudely, black ink on a torn piece of cardboard: "Found: Lady's Watch," and it too left a number.

That means, between Tuesday and Thursday morning—because when we ran on Tuesday we saw no signs and then ran Thursday and saw both—two different people had not only found watches but both felt compelled to track down their owners. One good running deed spawned another.

"I thought the watch was gone for good, but my wife told me that runners have a good spirit," says Jeremy Daveau, who had lost his Garmin—a gift for his fortieth birthday—on Wednesday morning and was reunited with it on Saturday night. When he went to visit Marie Bouvet and Peter Rainforth—the friends training for a triathlon who had posted the original message—he brought them a bottle of Champagne. "It speaks to who we are as human beings that if you find something that doesn't belong to you, you don't steal it, because you know that person needs it for their training," Daveau says. "They need it for their passion."

AT THIS STAGE of the game, my friend, you're a runner. Even if you haven't been following the program, haven't completed two races, don't do speed work, skip most of your long runs, and haven't even tried on your shoes for a while. If you're embarking on the half-marathon, let's face it: you run. But along with that title come certain responsibilities. Heavy is the crown.

In an article published in the *Wall Street Journal*, taken from a speech to graduating college seniors, economics professor Charles Wheelan wrote, "Don't make the world worse. I know that I'm supposed to tell you to aspire to great things. But I'm going to lower the bar here: just don't use your prodigious talents to mess things up. Too many smart people are doing that already." Are you doing your part? Let's say you see someone running—do you give them a nod, maybe say good morning, before moving on? Do you donate old shoes? Volunteer at races? And what about snot rockets? Before launching, do you first make sure the coast is clear?

"Years back, in the first running boom, runners were purely competitive, and I think today's runners do it to lose weight or socialize, and that's admirable," Bill Rodgers says. "I take my hat off to them, but the activity of running has overwhelmed the sport, and there's a certain unconsciousness among the newbies about our history and customs."

Like a lot of vets, Rodgers has forgone the marathon, but he still enjoys running the half. Today, a middle-of-the-pack runner, he has the opportunity to meet lots of first-time participants in the sport he helped popularize in the '70s. One thing that bugs him is the predominance of earphones, which he feels make people oblivious to other runners: "They used to have music at the finish line—and I love music, Stevie Wonder, Van Morrison—but you see it on the course, and it can be a pain in the you-know-what. It doesn't make sense to do an activity in the crowded public and lose your communication skills," says Rodgers. "You have people who want to pass!" (Interestingly, the Boston Marathon prohibits runners competing for prize money from listening to music, while the general public is allowed. Perhaps there really is an advantage to blasting Paul Simon's favorite songs.)

Clearly, as someone moving sky and earth to get music recommendations, I'm all for listening to music when you run. But there's an unwritten contract you sign by doing that: you have to stay conscious of where you are, who's around you, and who—like Bill Rodgers, the all-time victory leader at the World Marathon Majors—might want to pass. Already the New York City Marathon's "strongly discouraged" music players, and this is a horrible thing: it's fun to see yourself starring in your own action film, blasting Young Jeezy, Broken Social Scene, Selena Gomez, or Marilyn Manson, and finding motivation in your favorite tunes. However, you're not in your basement on a treadmill. You're outside, in public, near cars, in a crowded area: becoming oblivious is not only selfish, it's dangerous too.

A UNIVERSITY could be erected to teach all the customs we follow to become better runners, and none of them has anything to do with taking a minute or two off our time. The running world's a community, and like it or not, you're now a representative of that community. If you leave empty Gatorade bottles at the track or take a leak on someone's front lawn before a race, that's how runners behave. Whatever you do, that's what runners do, who runners are: so don't cuss out volunteers if they drop your water and don't run with your shirt off if you live on a crowded street with people eating outside. No one wants your sweat on their salad. What does the running world look like in 2014? Look in the mirror: the answer is you.

"About thirty years ago, there weren't that many runners, so everyone you passed would sort of nod and say hi," says Bert de Vries, who makes all of his Longboat Roadrunners volunteer at two races before they can join. "It used to be that if a guy didn't nod back at you, you knew he was American, but it's sort of like we're all Americans today."

One month before participating in a half-marathon in Las Vegas, I'm celebrating Thanksgiving with Budweiser, the New England Patriots, too much turkey, and my family in Denver, so even though I live in Toronto, I'm as American as Black Friday sales at Best Buy. Still, that doesn't offend me. De Vries is right. Of course, the reverse can be true—which a New Yorker told me is considered to be Midwesternish—runners can be overly friendly, overly engaging, a little too rah-rah for certain tastes. Kenneth Mungara doesn't want to talk about his children when he's at the starting line, and Deena Kastor, the American women's record-holder in both the marathon and half-marathon, is all for signing autographs—after she's done setting records, not before. Nod at other runners, keep track of your litter, and, if you're running in a pack, run single file. Before a race, use a port-a-potty, and, above all else, always stop if another runner needs help.

Here are seven key principles they could teach at the Grace University of Running:

1. Talk about running with your running friends; with everyone else, talk about your law degree.
2. When you're in a bar or, better, the Oval Office, don't stretch your diaphragm.
3. Wear your running clothes when you're running, not when you're out on a date.
4. Ask "How was your run?" not "What was your time?" Don't lose track of what matters.
5. If you're running on a path, don't speed up to overtake someone then slow down just a step before them. Also, if you're running with someone, don't suddenly decide to race at the

very end—if your opponent doesn't know that you're racing, you're not.

6. If a dog off a leash in a non-off-leash zone jumps at you, it's OK to give it a kick. Its owner is an asshole.

7. Don't cut a course, lie about your time, flake out on your partner, or fake an injury. Make the running community a place you'd want your daughter to be.

"I was on a running trail, training for an Ironman, getting ready for a twenty-mile run, and there was this guy on a bike that was really sketchy, creeping me out," says Jean Knaack, executive director of the Road Runners Club of America. Every time Knaack stopped, the guy on the bike stopped. Every time she sped up, he sped up too. Going out alone in the woods is a classic horror film setup, but that's exactly what runners do. Thankfully, runners, the real ones, act as our own Neighborhood Watch.

"I wasn't sure what I was going to do. Should I go home? Could I even get out? But then all of the sudden I saw this guy running toward me. He had that real runner look—he was even wearing a hat for a triathlon I'd run—and I stopped him and pointed out the guy, and this runner, a random stranger, ran with me for six miles, until the creepoid on the bike disappeared," Knaack recalls. She adds that this runner's code works the same way as rule number one when it comes to racing or training: if you see someone down, it's your duty to help. "Runners should know CPR because, although it's unlikely, if someone has a pre-existing cardiac problem, it can be exacerbated by strenuous exercise," Knaack says. "You don't pass by a fallen runner—even if you're racing. It's part of the oath you take by slapping on running shoes."

At the Scotiabank Toronto Waterfront Marathon in October, Reid Coolsaet and Eric Gillis, who train together in Guelph, were trying to hit the Olympic standard to reach the London Olympic Games. I like these guys, not only because they're Canada's best runners and when they're done training they join the rest of their team in two old garbage cans loaded with ice, but also because they're great examples of how to run—great examples of form.

Coolsaet finished his race in 2:10:55, his personal best, and a time that qualified him for the Olympics. On crossing the finish line, he turned around. He didn't celebrate. He stood at the wire, cheering on his friend. "It's not about running; it's in every aspect of life. Reid and I are training partners, and it's not surprising he was able to switch gears pretty quickly," says Gillis. All his life, Coolsaet dreamt of the Olympics, and at the very moment he qualified, he thought of his teammate.

Gillis responded. He ran as hard as he could through the tape and met the Olympic qualifying time, by one second. "Whether you're running in the Olympics or running around your block, all runners do the same thing," Gillis says. "You've got to tip your hat to them, congratulate them, and give them their due."

RUNNERS HAVE recently been put into extraordinary situations and responded heroically, with valor. It started at the 2011 New York City Marathon when runners who'd traveled from all over the world to compete in the bucket list race suddenly found themselves in the midst of the catastrophe left by Hurricane Sandy. What did they do? When the race was canceled, they helped out, donated money and supplies, and made their way, en masse, to Staten Island, where nineteen people had been killed in the community that serves as the marathon's starting point. The runners passed out energy bars and baby wipes, and dressed in their running gear to change peoples' perceptions of these entitled athletes, they assisted in cleaning up the mess. "We wanted to turn a negative into a positive," one runner told the *Huffington Post*. Then, of course, there is Boston. Selfless is a word rarely associated with the marathon and yet what are we to make of the runners who had just finished their race, turned around when the bombs struck, and headed straight into the carnage? More than one report mentioned how runners tore off their shirts to use as tourniquets on their fellow racers.

We're runners, sure, but we're also human beings. So to everyone running in memory of a loved one or raising money by running for a cause close to your heart, a round of applause. And thanks to all runners who helped out in Boston and New York. You make all of us look good. I'll give the last word to Kathrine Switzer: "When you're a runner—a real runner—you know anything can happen. That's why the best runners are appreciative, respectful, and helpful: we have to look after our own."

THE SOUNDTRACK: Metric

When I proposed to Julie, it was on a boat heading to Toronto Island to see a Broken Social Scene concert. We got off the ship, called our parents, and headed to the stage to watch Metric, then an opening act, perform. Metric, born and based in Toronto, was our favorite group and we danced and held hands and prepared for the rest of our lives. I've had the good fortune of covering Metric often as they've gone from openers to headliners on their own. The band is fronted by Emily Haines, a Canadian rocker who looks like Rooney Mara, wears knee-high boots when she performs in Ottawa, and can reduce a veteran music reporter to a little boy. I mentioned that fact in my last piece on the band, probably more than I needed to, and prompted an email from my father with the headline: Negative Blogs. I didn't mean to be disrespectful and I never apologized to Haines or the group, so here goes: Your music has probably changed our lives and it's certainly gotten us through many a difficult moment. I would never want to reduce you, and I'm sorry if that's what I did.

Naturally, Metric was the first group I asked for running songs and when I caught up with Haines and the band's guitarist and producer Jimmy Shaw—interviewed before playing a benefit show for Toronto's Centre for Addiction and Mental Health—they graciously picked a tune.

"Me going for a run, the only thing I listen to is a siren," says Shaw.

"One good one is EMA's 'California.' There's no beat, no motivational message, no leotard, but it is a complete Fuck You, which is always a great thing that makes me want to run," says Haines.

"For me it would be anything by T. Rex, even though it's slow. Their songs always make me motivated," says Shaw, "but I don't run—I do an hour and a half onstage."

To which Haines added, "That EMA track is pretty awesome."

17

KEEPING
THE PACE

THE TRAINING: Reaching the Magnificent 17K

WEEK 35: Two runs, one for 8K (5 miles) and one for 16K (10 miles), with a 35-minute rowing machine session (or swim or cycle) in between.

WEEK 36: Try 3 runs, 2 easy for 8K and one long run of 17K (10.5 miles). At this point, you're ready for the half!

THE SOUNDTRACK: Willie Nelson

THE FINISH LINE: The half, now just about 5 weeks away!

FOR THE NEXT two weeks, be mindful of how long it takes you to complete your long run so you get a sense of how long it might take you to finish your race. This is the essence of long-distance running: pacing, breathing, fueling, finding a reserve of strength, of inner strength, when you're tired, sore, and aching. Surprise yourself, be a fighter—running for 13K (8.1 miles) is something most people don't do. Take pride in your accomplishment. Take pride in making time even to attempt it. And during your long run this week, pay attention to your form and visualize yourself on race day. Another tool to keep running fresh is imagination: your house isn't your house, but a finish line, and there waiting is Lana Del Rey or Kris Kristofferson and all your cheering family and friends.

Next week, do 8K (5 miles) slowly and get plenty of rest, because you're attempting 17K (10.5 miles). That's the apex of your workout, the needle beyond which you can cross that half-marathon finish line. Spending time on the rowing machine, running fartleks, doing hill workouts, all of these will help you finish faster, but success is a result of rest, accumulating miles, and knocking off that 17K long run.

Time yourself on your 17K and work out your average per-kilometer pace. Now project your half-marathon finishing time by multiplying that number by 21.1. For instance, in 2012, the average female half-marathon finisher took 2:19:47 to finish, at an average pace of 6:35 per kilometer (10:36 per mile). That means, if she runs each kilometer at about the same speed, she'd be at 1:51:59 at 17K. Of course, as you run farther, it's harder to maintain your speed. What speed can you maintain for two hours? If you start thinking about this stuff before the race starts, you'll run with more confidence and be more likely to enjoy the experience and keep moving forward to the marathon. (Or, if it's enough that you're out there running and you don't want to crunch numbers, no worries.)

If you feel ambitious, run a half-marathon. Try your 11K (6.8-mile) route twice and see what happens. Sometimes I feel like we're too afraid. The first time I learned I could run long is when I was with my sister on a treadmill. She was running for an hour, and I just tried to keep up. I'd never been on a treadmill for an hour before, but because she was doing it, I did it too. Test yourself. Take chances. As always, the big rule of thumb is Don't Be Stupid. But you're not in a hamster cage. You're free.

REST WILL CURE almost everything: rest and stretches and the occasional restorative Scotch. It's all about finding a pace you can maintain. Mickey Hall had to teach that to his son. When Ryan came home from Stanford and wanted to drop out of college and quit running, the old man told the kid to slow down: "He was depressed and miserable. In high school, he won almost everything, but at Stanford, away from home where he couldn't get much rest, he thought training harder meant training better and he was doing too much and running too fast—and getting licked." Mickey Hall is a marathon runner, trainer, and Ironman veteran, who started the cross-country program at his son's high school in Big Bear, California, to find his boy someone to run with.

Ryan Hall, Mickey's kid, is America's fastest marathon runner, but at Stanford he had dropped his father's training program—which had been borrowed from the Kenyans—and began each workout with fifteen minutes of walking and started practice with (excruciating for elite athletes) seven-minute miles, a much slower pace than he wanted to go. "It's like holding back a wild stallion; he wants to go out and just blast it. But if you want to work on your speed, you need to work on the zones," says Hall, who would follow his son on his bicycle and pop up at various parts of his training route, testing his heart rate.

The idea behind a "zone workout" is to run aerobically for as long as possible, using oxygen rather than glycogen as fuel, and holding off on the anaerobic workout until you need to surge at the end of a race. If you switch to an anaerobic workout too early, you'll find you have nothing left as the marathon gets long. Even with proper fueling, glycogen is a finite resource, which is why we hit the Wall: we use too much too soon and have nothing in the tank—no glycogen—for the finish line.

"You see old marathoners getting better and running faster because they learn their correct pace," says Hall, pointing out that the men's marathon winner at the 1984 Summer Olympics was thirty-seven years old (and only started to get good as a distance runner at twenty-seven). The female winner at the 2008 Beijing Olympics was thirty-eight, the oldest Olympic marathon champion of all time. Reid Coolsaet crunched the numbers of the top sixteen male finishers at the London Olympics and discovered that the average marathoner hit his best time on the eighth try.

The 1984 Summer Olympics were held in Los Angeles, and Hall and his son drove down from Big Bear to watch the marathon. Mickey Hall says he had an epiphany while watching that race. "Less and less about running the marathon is about God-given talent," he says. "More and more, it becomes about conditioning, strategy, and pace."

Runners find their pace in different ways. Dick Beardsley is one of the world's most famous marathon runners, but he's best known for a race he didn't win and the events that followed. In 1982, he ran the Boston Marathon and, after miles of running neck and neck with Alberto Salazar, wound up finishing just two seconds behind him in an event that's become known as the Duel in the Sun. "Once we dropped Bill Rodgers on the lower Newton Hills, it was Alberto and I, and when we turned right on Commonwealth at seventeen miles, I was going to run as hard as I could up Heartbreak and then even harder back down it," says Beardsley, who's been running for thirty-nine years. He swears he's never put much stock in pacing; for him, running is just finding the race's fastest runner and sticking with him the whole time.

"We ran those four miles faster than anyone's ever run it. I'm flying down that last big hill, trying to shake him, but when I get to the bottom, he's still right there with me and I can't feel my legs! I say to myself: this isn't good." Nine hundred meters from the Boston Marathon finish line, Beardsley was winning and made his move: "I knew Alberto didn't have a great closing kick, but as I pushed off on my right leg to finish him, my hamstring cracked and Alberto took the lead." Beardsley was basically counted out as Salazar gained, and—you can see this on YouTube—the motorcade driving alongside the leaders began to coalesce around Salazar before the race was through. With six hundred meters to go, after running for more than twenty-six miles, Beardsley caught Salazar. "Alberto had gotten a hundred meters on me, but I just started flying—I don't remember my feet touching the ground," says Beardsley, who held on for a matter of seconds but then had to widen his route to the finish line to avoid a security guard on a bike and was unable to catch one of the running world's all-time biggest stars. "If I had gone slower earlier, would I have had more at the end? Hard to say, but I don't think so. Every race you run, every mile, is its own perfect thing."

What followed for Beardsley was a series of setbacks and accidents, addictions, and nightmares. Born and raised in Northern Minnesota, he spent his life around farms. On November 13, 1989, he got up as usual at 4 a.m. to milk his seventy cows, and then, somehow, while he was using an auger attached to his tractor to lift corn into a crib, his left leg got stuck in the drill.

"It wrapped me up to my groin and started taking my whole body, whipping me around, and I could feel myself losing consciousness. But if I went out, I knew it would be all over. By the grace of God, I made it to the lever to turn off the power. Next thing I know, I'm laying on the ground—my left foot sticking in my left ear." Beardsley had lived his whole life as a runner, but it seemed those days were through. "They tried putting my leg back together, but it was surgery after surgery, infection after infection, for years," he says, adding that having his leg nearly chopped off was tough; battling the ensuing painkiller drug addiction was nearly impossible. "They made that farm accident seem like a walk in the park. I was lying to my family, forging prescriptions. Those drugs are the devil, and it's a blessing, now that it's over and done with, that I'm still alive."

Today, Beardsley's clean, remarried, living in Austin, and once again running. He's currently up to 112 kilometers (70 miles) a week and, since 2000, has been running marathons, coming in under 2:50 more than once. "I love running today as much as I ever have. It's my little one-on-one time with the good Lord, and it helps me with my sobriety and everything else in my life," he says. "If I couldn't run, I'd be a cyclist, and if I couldn't cycle, I'd walk, and if I couldn't walk, I'd get out there on some kind of rowing machine. I like how it makes me feel."

It only feels good if you go at the right speed. If you're in the wrong French class, you're not going to like school. To make sure that his runners are paced correctly, Mickey Hall puts heart monitors on the entire Big Bear High track team, and every two weeks he has them trot across the same 5K (3-mile) training course on relatively flat terrain. If their heart rate goes above 130, the runners slow down. It's not about how fast they run; it's about keeping their heart rate down, pacing their bodies, and not burning glycogen. He's conditioning their hearts. "If my training is right, and the pacing is right, I'm expecting that each time I run the trial, the time will be quicker at the same heart rate," he says. "All we want is to see the aerobic speed improving. How fast can you run aerobically? In a race, whoever stays aerobic the longest will win."

For us, a successful half-marathon will just mean finishing without injury, but the Hall principles apply to everyday runners just as much as they do to the marathon world's stars. And, make no mistake, Hall has produced winners, though none more famous than that near-Stanford dropout, his son. Eventually, Ryan Hall returned to college, switched up his training, and became excited about running again. In 2008, he was America's second finisher in the Olympic marathon, taking tenth place overall. He's still the first American to run the half-marathon in less than an hour, and despite not finishing at the 2012 Olympic Games, he holds the fastest marathon time ever by an American, 2:04:58 at the 2011 Boston Marathon. His dad thinks he can go faster. It won't happen if he screws up his pace.

FINDING YOUR pace takes discipline, and this is where running becomes mystical. It's not only about running as fast as you can but also about running as fast as you can at a tempo you can sustain across miles and miles. Mike Austin teaches philosophy at Eastern Kentucky University and has written extensively on the mind games that go into distance training. "Something about the marathon attracts people who are introspective, sometimes morbidly so," says Austin, who recalls a time when he defaulted at a high school track meet and was told by his coach that he was "being selfish." By surrendering to his adrenaline, he was too immature to capitalize on his talent. The coach said: Grow up. "A lot of philosophers find value in acquiring self-knowledge, and there's parallels between self-knowledge and doling out energy over the course of a long run," Austin says, pointing out that marathon running is about balancing two contradictory compulsions: controlling yourself and letting go.

In 1985, Austin ran the St. Louis Marathon, and he still applies what he learned in that race to his everyday life. A father of three teenage girls, he knows certain behaviors push his buttons, just like he knows he tends to run too quickly at the start of a race. But by being aware of these tendencies, he guards against his initial impulses and is able to exert self-control. Self-control, that which separates adults from children, is discussed in great detail in *Willpower*, a book by psychologist Roy Baumeister and science writer John Tierney. In the book, they suggest discipline works like a muscle and can become stronger the more that it's used. However, like any muscle, it also has its limits and can snap.

As you feel yourself getting faster, you might be tempted to run much more often. Don't do it. You need to find the sweet spot where you're gradually going just a little bit farther at a sustainable speed. It's better to get stronger, not weaker, as you get deeper into a race: no one cares who was winning a half-marathon at 8K.

THE SOUNDTRACK: Willie Nelson

Willie Nelson is one of those people you wish you could sit beside on a long plane ride. He's had four wives, been rich and poor, and has played the same guitar, "Trigger," named after Roy Rogers's horse, since 1969. What hasn't he seen in his lifetime?

Now eighty, Nelson mentions that he has just earned his second-degree black belt in tae kwon do. He says, "I run too, but a lot of times when I'm out there, I'm not listening to music, I'm listening to hear if I'm still breathing... I take my iPhone with me sometimes on a run, and I'm probably just listening to some [Kris] Kristofferson or Hank Williams." Although he's covered both Pearl Jam and Coldplay on recent albums, he reveals that bands like that come to him through the recommendation of his sons.

Nelson's also made two songs with Snoop Dogg—"We met in Amsterdam," he tells me—but when pressed for a selection from Snoop's catalog, he switches the conversation back to Kristofferson and Hank.

"I'll recommend 'Help Me Make It Through the Night,' and 'Loving Her Was Easier (Than Anything I'll Ever Do Again)' by Kristofferson and 'Hey, Good Lookin',' 'Move It On Over,' and 'Jambalaya' by Hank Williams."

I asked Willie why these songs would be good for running, and he mentioned their exquisite composition, lyrics, and energy. "These are just some of my favorite songs," he says. "They've kind of grown on me after almost fifty years of playing them every night."

18

101 WAYS TO KICK HALF-MARATHON ASS

THE TRAINING: Mixed Taper

WEEK 37: Do 1 run of 10K (6 miles). For your second workout, spend 30 minutes on a bike, in a pool, or using a rowing machine. Finally, run 8K (5 miles), slowly.

WEEK 38: Take 3 runs, each no farther than 5K (3 miles) and do everything super slowly.

THE SOUNDTRACK: The Cranberries, Moby, The Gaslight Anthem, The National, and Joan Baez

THE MENU: Gordon Ramsay

THE FINISH LINE: The half, now just 3 weeks away.

WE'VE COVERED a lot of ground to get to race day, but this is probably the most important thing you'll read: ninety-six hours from the start line, don't run. When the half is three weeks away, try something like 10K (6 miles) with a cross-training session and another 8K (5 miles) mixed in. Two weeks out, you might run 5K (3 miles) a few times, or take another ride on the bike, but do everything slow and easy. You've already done so much—it's time to put up your feet. Here are 101 other tips for enjoying your half-marathon.

1. Don't do anything before the race or during the race that you haven't already done in practice.
2. And before race day, please know what you're going to wear, what you're going to eat, and how you're going to get to the race... please?
3. "Look like a bum, run like a bum," says Duff McLaren, who has run fifty-one marathons. What he means is, wear something special on race day.
4. Even if it's just lucky socks, I might add. Whatever you think works, works.
5. Except, honor tradition. Don't wear your race shirt on race day. Run the race first—that shirt must be earned.
6. This, from Gordon Ramsay, who has run the marathon twice: "A simple pasta with a tomato base as a pre-marathon meal for energy. A quick carb hit beforehand; you don't want anything too fancy. For afterward, a nice simple steak and a salad to take in some protein to start the process of repairing muscles."
7. He also said: "Never race against your wife!" (In London, his wife, Tana, overtook him at Mile 21 and beat him by fifteen minutes.)
8. If you're comfortable before the race starts, you're dressed too warmly.
9. Wear something disposable to the starting line—like a trash bag.
10. And, guys, avoid shaving on race day—the aftershave gets in your eyes.
11. Suntan lotion does, too. If you think it's going to be sunny, wear a hat.

12. A white one, eh? And, if you're traveling to a race, bring these things.

13. Don't buy stuff at the race expo, the giant shopping mall you have to walk through to pick up your bib, and then wear it in the race untried.

14. See Rule No. 1.

15. Also, don't try to pick up your packet on race-day morning. That's the busiest time of the entire event and absolutely certain to be a clusterfuck.

16. Equally important: stash your postrace bag with a friend or hide it somewhere in the woods. Avoid the postrace baggage claim like a lawyer.

17. You don't need to bring a giant water belt. You're an athlete now, so pick up your water on the run.

18. Noel Hogan, guitarist for The Cranberries, recommends *Rearviewmirror* by Pearl Jam and "Disarm" by the Smashing Pumpkins. "I can't run without music," he says. "If my batteries die, the run starts to feel really long." You're about to run the half-marathon. Even with your batteries charged, it's going to feel really long. Why not charge your batteries?

19. Men, smear petroleum jelly under your arms and on your nipples. Women, it goes between your thighs and sometimes around the bra line. It's just as important as shoes are.

20. Also, pace bands are available on lots of websites and at every good sneaker store. These bracelets list split times for every kilometer (or mile) based on your expected finish. You'll probably ignore these times. Wear one anyway.

21. And you haven't trained for thirty-nine weeks and then forgotten to double-knot your laces.

22. Double-knot your laces!

23. When the gun goes off, go crazy: scream, cheer, yell. You're alive!

24. But then use the 1K (or 1-mile) marker as a sign to settle down. There's no way you can sustain that kind of intensity.

25. But I'm serious, get into it: there are few things as thrilling as the start of a race.

26. Remember, this is fun.

27. So go easy on the water. It's a half-marathon in the city, not 100 miles through the desert. The winner's rarely the one who has to stop the most to pee.

28. Moby has a few suggestions for what you should be listening to...

29. "Will the Circle Be Unbroken" by John Lee Hooker.

30. "Strange Fruit" by Billie Holiday.

31. "Damaged I" by Black Flag.

32. But even if you are listening to Moby's suggestions, don't listen to music throughout the whole race. When else in life do you get to hear people cheering you on?

33. And take a minute to scope out the other runners. The half's a lot easier when you find someone to run with.

34. So don't look at your watch too much. It's much more fun to look at the crowd.

35. Thank the volunteers. You want to encourage people to keep doing this, right?

36. Also, there's no better feeling on earth than high-fiving a kid. Be kind to the next generation of runners.

37. If you really, really, really need to pee, just do it. It's uncomfortable holding it the whole time.

38. Just think about reaching 5K. Wipe everything else from your mind.

39. At 4K (2.8 miles), exhale: you're just about through that first wild bit. Coast for a minute, relax.

40. Doesn't that water taste good? Make sure you're drinking. Don't go overboard—this isn't a cruise ship. But the idea is to

drink BEFORE you get thirsty (and you don't need a whole lot, sometimes just a sip will do).

41. Gatorade can get rid of cramps, which are a result of dehydration. Sports drinks send electrolytes into the bloodstream faster than regular old H_2O.

42. Resist early overconfidence. If you feel great, awesome, ride that, but don't mistake that feeling for licking the run.

43. Races begin near the finish line—30K (18.6 miles) in the marathon, 15K (9.3 miles) in the half.

44. That's why it's good to chomp on race gels. Just be certain to sample one during practice if you're going to use them in a race. Some are hard to swallow and might make you nauseous—as a rule of thumb, see Rule No. 1.

45. Otherwise, pop a gel or an energy chew every 5K. It will give you a boost when you take one—and when you spend the rest of the time thinking about how good it will feel when you take one again.

46. If your energy chews come individually packaged, unwrap them before the race and put them in a resealable plastic bag. They'll melt in the heat, so in warm weather, forget about these gummies and try the jamlike gels.

47. And no offense, but if you're running with a friend and your friend is slower than you are, lose 'em. This is race day, not some rinky-dink training run.

48. That said, you shouldn't really be racing until you're at least halfway.

49. So toe a straight line—no curvy stuff. Twenty-one kilometers (13.1 miles) is long enough without adding any extra distance. Save the zigzags for after the race.

50. When you feel like you can't go on, control your breathing. Your breath is the key to your rhythm. Control your breath; control your body—breathe.

51. There's absolutely nothing wrong with walking. The thing you're fighting against is giving up.
52. At 10K (6 miles), acknowledge the achievement. You're going to do this; you're doing it. You'll never be at this moment again.
53. You don't have to race, but you should have a time goal. Don't fall asleep out there. Keep pressing. Keep pushing. Just focus on making it halfway.
54. Think negative split, or running the second half of your race faster than your first.
55. Basically, what I'm saying is push yourself, but save something for the end.
56. It's hard and I can rarely do it, the negative split, I mean—but that doesn't mean you shouldn't try.
57. Stick to your race plan!
58. When you hit the halfway mark, start counting the kilometers down instead of up. It feels like ticking off the final seconds on New Year's Eve.
59. Seriously, when you're halfway, smile. Don't make it bigger than it is. Remember, you paid; you're not being paid. It's very unlikely, no matter how well you do, that you'll win.
60. That said, if you don't sleep the night before the race, don't worry. It's two nights before the race that's important.
61. Pre (the legendary Steve Prefontaine) never slept the night before a big race. And he's like Rihanna, so famous in running that he only went by one name. Want some inspiration? Watch just about any documentary about the man and get pumped for your race.
62. Race! At some point during the second half of your half-marathon, push. You are wearing a race bib after all: experiment with leaving your comfort zone.
63. Flex. Psychologically, I mean. Get tough. The half-marathon isn't for the faint of heart, which is good because you're not faint of heart. Remind yourself of that again and again.

64. Brian Fallon, leader of The Gaslight Anthem, says "Audience" by Cold War Kids helps him flex psychologically. "It's forward-moving music and has a beat you can follow that pushes you. It gets me psyched. If I was a runner, this is what I'd listen to."

65. Still, try not to put your music on until you hit 15K. Keep it in your pocket like a secret weapon.

66. I like to think I'm like a boxer who has fought the whole match southpaw, but really I'm a rightie. Then, at 15K, I turn on my music—and suddenly, Rocky-style, I'm fighting with the proper hand.

67. Ryan Hall, whom you've met, says, "Pray. Ask God what you should do. God knows you and knows your body and knows exactly what would be best for you. He usually wakes me up in the night and gives me some brilliant ideas."

68. Hall also practices lots and lots.

69. Which means there's no such thing as a race-day miracle. Manage your expectations: what you ran in practice is probably pretty close to what you'll run in the race.

70. Always, always, always, always keep your head up in a race.

71. And let other runners block the wind for you. The only time you need to be ahead of someone else is at the finish line.

72. When you need a burst of speed, exaggerate your arm swing.

73. And when you get tired, concentrate on lifting your knees.

74. And it always helps me to keep my head in a race by lengthening my stride. Technically, this is not considered great form because it can lead to overstriding and injury, but whatever works, right? Many people now suggest putting your hands above your head to reset your form, i.e., to get your feet below your hips, or picking up your cadence. So, if you find lengthening your stride feels weird, pretend you're at a rock show and lift up your hands.

75. When the finish line gets to within single digits, that's your cue to pick up your speed.

76. Or, if your race is more about survival, when the finish gets to within single digits, that's your cue—you will survive.

77. Even when you're exhausted, don't cut people off at the water stations and try not to bean anyone with your cup.

78. That said, if shit happens, don't be a baby. Races are weird, and weird things happen. Simon Whitfield, a Canadian triathlete, was competing in the 2000 Athens Olympics when he crashed his bike. Fourteen riders went down. Whitfield picked himself up and kept riding. "Pretty much after that happened I threw caution to the wind," he says. "I was excited as I kept passing people, but honestly? I never expected to win gold."

79. "I ran yesterday for the first time since high school," says Matt Berninger, singer of The National. "I couldn't walk for three days." What was he listening to? *I Care Because You Do* by Aphex Twin. "But I had to stop before the record was over and crawl home," he says.

80. A mantra or chant can help spur you on when you feel like Matt Berninger. Joan Benoit Samuelson, winner of the 1984 Olympic women's marathon, repeats the names of her children. If you feel yourself wavering, repeat the name of someone you love.

81. You might also write down their name or an inspiring word or catchphrase on your arm.

82. It's OK to stop and take a picture. It's a mortal sin to stop and talk on the phone.

83. You've been knocking off 8K on your easy runs. When you get down to eight during the race, be confident: you've been here before.

84. Know the terrain. Where are the hills? Where are the turns? Where's the finish line?! Don't let the race catch you by surprise.

85. Which is why it's important to listen to the race chatter. What are people saying about the wind? The heat? The party after? Gather information like a twenty-year-old web billionaire.

86. It's nice to make friends.

87. When Joan Baez can't find inspiration on the treadmill, she listens to "Bamboleo" by The Gypsy Kings. She says, "Somehow it gets into my bones."

88. Which brings up a good point. When programming your music, it's not about speed but spirit. My No. 1 favorite desert island running pick of all time? Paul Simon's "Graceland." Neil Diamond's "I Am I Said" is a close No. 2. And Bad Brains' "I Against I" comes in third.

89. At 17K (10.5 miles), give someone in the crowd a high-five. You're about to finish doing something you've never done before.

90. So encourage other runners around you. Let good vibes be what the race remembers you for.

91. If you have a problem and feel like you can't go on, move off to the side.

92. Your only goal right now should be to finish. Until race day, no one knows how fast they are.

93. Truthfully, sometimes the only thing you can do is hold on.

94. Clench and unclench your fists if you're exhausted, stay straight, and take off that iPod. With 2K (1.4 miles) left, damn right you want to be listening to the people on the streets.

95. This is the climax of your movie. What happens to the hero is all up to you.

96. And it's OK to yell when you're digging down deep. This isn't a dinner party, and you're not at church. Scream your head off as you dip into your last leg: this is what you paid your entrance fee for.

97. When you see the finish line, go like hell.

98. At the moment of truth, try mustering a smile. This is where the photographs are taken, and, despite the exorbitant prices, you'll probably still buy the damn thing.

99. Don't stop when you cross the line. Others will be pouring in behind you, so keep walking. This will also help keep the sore muscles at bay.

100. Let a volunteer drape you in a medal, and eat all the free bagels and bananas you can.

101. What you've done is an accomplishment. However you've finished, you finished. You've won.

19

RACE THREE, RUNNING FREE: LAS VEGAS

MY FASTEST KILOMETER at the Rock 'n' Roll Las Vegas Marathon and Half-Marathon is from corral number forty-eight to the starting line. The gun's about to go off on Las Vegas Boulevard at the Mandalay Bay at what's being touted as the largest nighttime running event in the world. Like that's a good thing...

Some of the runners are dressed up as Elvis, forty-one people are getting married, and one man is wearing a pink gorilla suit. My goal's to run 1:30 for the half-marathon, but I've picked up on the fact that most people don't go to Vegas to achieve a personal best (PB) time: the guy beside me in the corral is warming up with a tallboy of Coors.

Kicking around the area a day before start time, I meet runners and explore the race expo at the Sahara. Expos are where the world comes together to sell shit to runners and it's neat to see all the different shoes and weird odds and ends that are out there. It's a good place to learn about farflung races and the latest compression socks, but it's a dangerous place to go shopping. Just collect the free samples, browse, and mingle with everyone else wearing yellow shoes.

Increasingly, people are participating in events out of town, turning a race into an active vacation. I tend to get anal and ruin the enjoyment—associating anything against a clock with a war—but that's not necessarily the right vibe. People are dressed up as Elvis for chrissakes. Usually that's a sign that the war is through. "It's fun here because you kind of forget that you're running," says a waitress at Serendipity 3, outside Caesars Palace. "It's like, you're just in Vegas and then—oh yeah, there's that run!"

I'm not quite that casual about it: even though I'm in Vegas, everything I eat, everything I do, everything I wear, is centered on my run. It's the beginning of December, and I'm registered for Boston in April—my half is a pivotal moment: it separates everything that's come before it from what's about to come next.

THE MORNING BEFORE the evening race is uneventful. Like an asshole, I jog the Strip, going up and down the steps to the different hotels, and pass a guy with a cigarette and a glass of wine and quite possibly a freezer full of bodies under his house. It's 7 a.m., and he tries to give me five as I run right past him in my ultra-lightweight Adidas Feathers. It's not yet breakfast time in Las Vegas, and here I am in pink sneakers with Vaseline on my nipples, and I make myself laugh: Esme's ear infection is important; my last training run in Sin City is not.

Still, I walk through The Bellagio with my kilometer split times on my hand. My leg hasn't bugged me since the fifteenth of November, and although I haven't really been training, I'd like to beat the 1:29 I ran in Oakville, just because.

At the start of any race I've come to expect pandemonium, but this is unreal. Of the 44,000 people participating in the Rock 'n' Roll Las Vegas Marathon and Half-Marathon,

38,000 are running the half. And that number's probably not even accurate. I've heard plenty of reports about people who signed up for the marathon and then, after a few days on the Strip, switched to the half. Some people just can't handle Vegas, I guess.

I make my way to my starting corral, and as Mike McCready, Pearl Jam's guitarist, plays "The Star-Spangled Banner," I take off and don't stop running until I reach corral number one. It's 10°C (50°F), evening, and I'm wearing shorts, shirt, jacket, lucky socks, and a hat. I meet an old man from Saskatoon who's run sixty-three marathons. He tells me I'm going to be warm.

Three kilometers (1.9 miles) in, it turns out the old man was right. I'm running at about pace, taking in surroundings that I've previously only seen at bachelor parties, and I feel a sense of relief that it's finally race time. Running is simple. Justifying going to Vegas for a half-marathon and leaving my wife with a sick newborn is hard. But soon enough, my mind is clear except for the hypnotic, addictive rhythm of my running. My body feels good, endorphins are firing, and I envision myself as electric as one of these neon signs.

We've passed Las Vegas Boulevard's good side at 5K (3 miles) and head into an underbelly on Main Street, which turns into Fourth Street and then Third Street and then Sixth. One of the best parts of running is that you get to explore, and we pass the pawn shops you don't see on TV. The locals are not your typical race fans—it's night, in Vegas, in the bad part of town—but they applaud nevertheless. The spectators may smoke and scream and raise Styrofoam cups, but they're still applauding. We trade nods and I clap for the people clapping for the race.

Night runs are inherently challenging; they're best for a unique experience, less than ideal for clocking a terrific time.

I can't lie. I only chose this race because I was invited and put up in a room. With night runs, it's difficult to know what to do with yourself on race day, and I can't quite find an edge. You need something extra when you're racing: an anger, a hunger, a desperation, a spark. That's tough to find after you've been floating in the Roman baths at Caesars Palace, and after forty-five minutes of running, past the halfway point, my concentration wanders and I vow to do a better job back at home. A little bit of guilt joins me for the rest of my run. The feeling isn't entirely unpleasant. I feel confident as I often do in my sneakers: challenges become possibilities. And it's almost like I'm mentally writing in my journal or else sightseeing on a tour bus when, quite naturally, I run into a friend. Together, we fall into an easy pace, something like 4:10 per kilometer (6:42 per mile), and he invites me to a party at Planet Hollywood later that night. I like him—he's Ken Riess, an exercise science professor at the University of Alberta—and we burn a few kilometers together until he starts getting tired, and I pop an energy gel and decide, OK, time to run.

Unfortunately, my body has other ideas. At 15K (9.3 miles), my time's 58:22. To hit 1:30, I'd only need to be at 1:03:59. But here's the thing about mental lollygagging and pacing: I sprint leaving Ken, but, with 5K left, my spirit leaves me. The distance between the Sahara and Mandalay Bay is only a bit more than 6K (4 miles), but I can't fuel a proper leg kick to attack the end of the race. There are no injuries, no cramps, I'm just feeling heavy, and thus a negative attitude encroaches. Instead of getting heated up, I become resigned. I don't even care about fighting anymore.

I bop down the Boulevard, passing the Encore Wynn, Bally's, and the MGM Grand, but I'm not particularly soaring with emotion. I can't find my fifth gear. People are imbibing on the sidelines, and there's almost a Mardi Gras vibe. But for all I know, this has nothing to do with the race—it's nighttime in Vegas, Mardi Gras all the time. I do not absorb any energy as I pound past the finish line.

Is it possible to run a lazy half-marathon? I come in at 1:28:40, beating my time in Oakville, and earning a new PB. Racing is a curious endeavor: I feel like I could've gone faster, but I ran faster than I'd ever run before. I go to a restaurant with some Canadians and have beer and steak, and more beer and steak, and celebrate my run. It's going to feel good to get home to Toronto. Sometimes the best part about doing something is when that something is done.

FOUR

BREAKING BARRIERS

THE

MARATHON

"I take what I do seriously.
I don't go out there to fuck around."

MATT LOISELLE, Canadian Olympic hopeful, with
apologies to his father, on how he prepares for the marathon

BOTTLING THE RUNNER'S HIGH

▬▬▬▬▬

THE TRAINING: Once More with Gusto

WEEK 40: Rest for a week after completing your half-marathon and enjoy all the Chinese food, margaritas, and sponge cake you earned.

WEEK 41: Run 8K (5 miles) once, spend 40 minutes rowing (or swimming or cycling), and start your long run, my friend, at 16K (10 miles).

THE SOUNDTRACK: The Black Keys, and a Katy Perry story about methodology

THE FINISH LINE: The marathon, now just about 13 weeks away.

CONGRATULATIONS ON completing your half-marathon, but now is the part of your training when things start to suck. The running's about to get (more) tough, time-consuming, and expensive. It might appear to your loved ones that there's someone new in your life. Your muscles will ache, causing you to limp up—and worse, down—your steps, and you'll probably become somewhat of a jackass as you insist to whomever will listen that you can't do whatever they're proposing because it's absolutely essential that you not miss a run. Here's the trick: Become insufferable as you prepare for the marathon so that you don't suffer as much when you run.

Of the four distances that we've trained for, the marathon's the least popular—by far. Flip to Chapter 13 for a taste of what it might feel like. And that was during a Boston Marathon-qualifying run. However, you don't need to run the marathon distance in practice to run that far in a race. Just as you ran 17K (10.5 miles) then completed the half-marathon, Dr. Ralph Vernacchia, director of the Center of Performance Excellence at Western Washington University and the co-chair of the USA Track and Field Psychology Sub-committee, says if you can get your long run up to 30K (18 miles or so), you can complete the marathon. At that point, the race becomes a mind game. "Marathon runners need to understand the cumulative effect of their training programs. Their performance depends on the total amount of miles they log before the marathon, not one or two long runs," Dr. Vernacchia says. That's why, in these next thirteen weeks of training, we're going to slowly increase the distance of the long run, but also augment these workouts with bi- or even tri-weekly speed work, cross-training, and slow 8 to 10K (5- to 6-mile) recovery runs. "To complete the marathon, it's the miles you run week to week that are essential. I've coached runners for twenty years, and consistent training and adherence to pacing—not a long run of more than 29K—are the keys to completing the marathon."

From here on in, each week's long run moves up 3K (1.9 miles), then drops back down every other week to let you rest. Your long run will top out at 30K (18.6 miles) at Week 49, three weeks out from race day. And for the next six weeks, you're going to stay with three workouts, but then we're going to build in a fourth. The idea for these weeks is to build mileage and slowly increase the distance of your long run. These numbers can be tweaked, and, as ever, mix in walking as you see fit, but the goal's to bring down the amount of time you walk. Record your results and, if you have to skip something, don't skip your long run. It's what gets you to the marathon.

Also, and this is essential, according to Dr. Vernacchia as important as or even more important than anything else, you need to be well rested when you approach the marathon starting line. Two weeks before the marathon, you'll only do 60 percent of your usual training mileage, then you'll drop to 30 percent the week before the big race.

At this point, you have to measure your distances. It's fine if you don't care about your time and just want to finish, but you need to keep track of how far you're running in practice. The average female marathon finisher is thirty-six years old and requires 4:42:10 to get across the finish line. The average guy's almost forty and needs 4:16:14. Know what to expect when you register. However, there are truths to be gleaned by running long distances, and one is the runner's high, the sport's holy grail.

THERE ARE LOTS of things about running that Josphat Nzinga didn't like. He had been a champion sprinter since the age of thirteen in Kathiani, Eastern Kenya, but aspects of the sport had grown tiresome. For one, when he raced against athletes from other townships, everyone just took off like mad at the starting gun, leaving little room for strategy and reducing the sport to one mad dash of four hundred or eight hundred meters—a quarter or halfway around the track. As he grew older, his body was too small to compete against the giants who seemed to have more power in each leg than he could muster from his entire scrawny frame.

In Kathiani, where Nzinga grew up without electricity or hot water, every kid's a runner, and he had been scuttling across his parents' farm barefoot or in hand-me-down sneakers since he was eight and ran 20K (12.8 miles) to and from school every day. He excelled at short distances but was losing his faith in the sport. Then sea change struck Kathiani. In 1993, Cosmas Ndeti, Josphat's uncle, won the Boston Marathon. For a village of three thousand people with no television or automobiles, the prize money and sponsorship swag that flowed through the neighborhood changed everything. Distance running, they realized, could make you rich.

"Everyone started to call me by my uncle's name," says Nzinga, who has a calm, easy manner like a lot of great Kenyan runners and professional athletes who expel minimal energy at everything other than that one thing that takes all they have. (In my home, he gravitates toward the baby the way most of my friends seem to be summoned unconsciously to the fridge for a beer—which, of course, Nzinga's never tried.) His uncle told him to forget about sprinting and take up the marathon. Then Cosmas Ndeti won the Boston Marathon in 1994 and 1995 and, for twelve years straight, was the fastest marathoner in the world.

In selling the sport to his skeptical nephew, Ndeti introduced a crazy concept: he said that running gets easier, not harder, the farther you go. "He would talk to me about how sometimes you're so comfortable that you don't even know you're going 26 miles, that it reaches a point where you're taking it easy; your body isn't doing anything. From the outside, people go 'Wow, he's running so fast!' but for you the running's almost like sleep," says Nzinga, who went on to train for the marathon with his cousin in Nairobi and slowly came to understand what his idol had meant.

He says his uncle spoke of the "dreamlike" effect of long-distance running, but that as a child, he didn't put much stake in the old man's words. How could you race to school and back in front of millions of people for impossible money and not feel like you were carrying the weight of the world? "He'd say that it reaches a point of stillness—your body isn't doing anything and you feel like you can fly," says Nzinga. "If you're not training enough, my uncle'd say that you can't bring your mind to that point, which is why people quit in the beginning. But if you train for the marathon properly, you'll feel like you're not running—even when you're pushing so hard."

IT'S TIME to concentrate on the marathon, and as you become self-obsessed and geek out about your fartleks and strides, remember that there's a reward beyond the medal that you'll get when it's over. It's called the runner's high, and it's the euphoric buzz that'll hit you as you become stronger, sometime around the two-hour mark as you run. "We were able to show the release of endogenous opiates into the brain," says Dr. Henning Boecker, a neurologist at Germany's Bonn University and one of the world's foremost authorities on the runner's high. "Opiates are used as painkillers—opium is derived from endogenous opiates—and this runner's high sensation is not only euphoria creating, but also pain inhibiting. We know there are marathon runners who do not feel any pain when they run."

Boecker is a cyclist and a half-marathon runner. A father of two, he conducts his experiments on Sigmund Freud Street and is making it his life's work to map out running's transcendent ability to draw pleasure from pain. In his research, conducted in Munich in 2006 with ten half-marathon runners, Boecker and his colleagues injected radioactive tracers into the brain of their subjects to block opioid receptors. The working theory, which proved to be true, was that if they injected opioids into the runners' brains after a two-hour run, the tracers would decrease in volume after the subjects produced new opioids on their own. He explains that it's like trying to fit a key into a lock: if the brain produces opiates after running, the receptors will be blocked and the injected material won't bind.

"The nice thing about it is it not only allows you to see if it happens, but it also allows you to see where in the brain this occurs," explains Dr. Boecker, who discovered that the runners' release of opioids occurred in the frontolimbic brain region, the area of the brain that controls our emotions. "I think future research will help us understand these mechanisms with regard to depression and the treatment of patients with chronic pain," Boecker says.

So what does this mean for you? Think of it as a chest bump from God while you're training. It's important to rest for a week after completing your half-marathon, but once you get back into it—Week 41 for anyone still trucking along from day one—run 8K (5 miles) once, to loosen up your muscles. Then, return to cross-training. I still think the rowing machine is the best non-running exercise for runners, so try to spend forty minutes on a rowing machine or else the same amount of time swimming or cycling. The long run begins at 16K, just about ten miles, which is a good base for getting started. For the average runner, this distance should take about two hours. You'll be tired, absolutely, but also remember what Boecker proved on Sigmund Freud Street: it's a neurological fact that running long distances makes you feel good. It changes the brain's chemistry, and that feeling—the runner's high—has been described as resembling everything from euphoria to a sense of weightlessness to being on drugs.

I've never confused marathon running with tripping out at a Diplo set on New Year's Eve, but sometimes I do reach a point on my long runs where I feel like I can run around the world. Like Cosmas Ndeti, I get comfortable, and even if I'm not stoned exactly, I'm in some sort of state of tranquility. I look at Esme, who at five months is now sleeping and rolling over, and I can see that the runner's high is a similar breakthrough. It's a weight off my shoulders, momentum, an "aha" moment, a positive sign that I'm doing OK, but it's also a neurological sensation that acts like a natural prescription pill whose limits are yet to be fully understood.

"Nobody thinks you can cure Alzheimer's with running," says Boecker, "but we're interested in using the body's own properties as a prevention of negative health."

ED WHITLOCK is a stubborn eighty-three-year-old man who's rail thin, has long white hair, and is almost always the smartest guy in the room. He holds most of the world's senior running records. In 2011, he was disappointed when it took him 3:15:54 to complete the Scotiabank Toronto Waterfront Marathon. To put Whitlock's achievement in context, 3,958 people ran the 42.195-kilometer course. He came in 296th. Only one guy was older—he was 101, and it took him nine hours to finish.

Whitlock's training is simple: every day, he runs the same three-hour loop through his local cemetery. "I don't suffer from those delusions that all this stuff happens magically. If I could do the marathon without training, I'd be all for that," says Whitlock, who broke a rib fetching his morning paper four weeks after scoring his 3:16 and spent a month having to sleep sitting up. The incident derailed his 2012 running goals. Instead of racing in April, he ran his next marathon, at age eighty-one, in the fall and finished in 3:30. If Whitlock had wanted to qualify for Boston, he'd have beaten his time by an hour and a half.

"I always tell this joke," Whitlock says. "If you're an athletic coach and want to find out if you have a good marathon prospect, shine a flashlight in his ear. If you can see light on the other side, odds are you have a good prospect." What he's saying is: don't expect the runner's high to do the work for you. There's voodoo out there in sneakerland, but the only way to unlock it is to repeat some variation of the Whitlock Method: run around in circles, over and over again.

DR. RICHARD RAWSON, associate director of the UCLA Integrated Substance Abuse Programs, however, is working with methamphetamine addicts and trying to replace the high they achieved from drugs with the sensation that comes from exercise. "Why does the brain respond to opiates with this tremendously strong reaction? There must be a neurological function," explains Dr. Rawson, by way of introducing the 1976 discovery of endorphins, the brain's natural painkillers, which were first identified by studying the effects of methadone for the treatment of addiction to heroin. These initial studies won Roger Guillemen and Andrew Schally a Nobel Prize—and they fuel Rawson's work today.

"Over the last ten years, it's been clinically proven that the runner's high changes mood and can treat depression and anxiety," says Rawson, who's halfway through a five-year study on addiction and relapse and attempting to treat dysphoria by using exercise to naturally alter the chemistry of an addicted mind. "We're interested in sustained mood elevation. So far, we like what we see."

The UCLA study involves 150 patients—Rawson's tested seventy-five so far—and after putting addicts through an eight-week trial of three-times-a-week exercise, he's certain this type of intervention can work. "We see mood differences, but also cognitive improvement—they think better and exhibit a better variety of memory and concentration functions," Rawson tells me, adding that his preliminary findings have shown that addicts who stick with an exercise program are 20 percent less likely to relapse. Of course, running a marathon isn't like slamming heroin or smoking a bowl of methamphetamine. Rawson says that on a euphoria scale of one to ten, if heroin takes you to a twelve, exercise may take you to a six. However, it can help rebuild neurotransmitters damaged by drug abuse and replace brain chemicals that have been sucked dry from drugs. "Addicts in recovery not only don't have the drugs they used, but they've damaged their baseline chemistry and feel depressed," says Dr. Rawson. "The idea that you can change this feeling—life sucks—with something other than an external drug is an empowering piece of knowledge."

FOR ALL practical purposes, you're probably not going to feel a runner's high as intense as that of a Kenyan three-time winner of the Boston Marathon or get as low as someone whose brain is recovering from an addiction to meth. Better you just tuck the runner's high away in your jacket pocket and think of it as a sign along the journey that you're getting close to your goals. Like most of us, consider it a feeling of accomplishment mixed with a certain giddiness in acknowledging that you're improving at something that's important to you. I always think about the marathon in these terms: there are so many things out there that I can't do. But then I try a long run, complete it—finish, succeed. You can too.

"HONESTLY, THE biggest thing for me in terms of euphoria is weather," says Lesley Taylor, our voice of running reason, who recently completed the New York City Marathon in 4:36. "When it's freezing and there's snow all over, I'm bitching the whole time. There's nothing enjoyable about it— no runner's high."

Josphat Nzinga, however, begs to differ. After leaving his career as a sprinter, he got serious about training for the marathon. It was hard at first, as expected—he'd become winded at two hours and wasn't used to not being the fastest one of his friends. But eventually, he turned a corner and finally he experienced his uncle's sense of weightlessness for himself. In 2011, he took first place at the Mississauga Marathon. You'll know when the runner's high hits you. It's when you forget that you're running at all.

THE SOUNDTRACK: The Black Keys
At an overpriced restaurant on the waterfront in Toronto, I meet Dan Auerbach and Patrick Carney, The Black Keys. The guys are enjoying a moment, or at least trying to, as they released *El Camino* and suddenly went from a popular indie rock band to the type of group that plays stadium shows.

"Just for the record, this isn't the kind of place that we usually hang out in," says Auerbach. "We don't hang out in spots that have $10 beers."

"Yeah," says Carney. "We usually hang out at the Ritz-Carlton and have $20 beers and Champagne."

The guys are not runners. In fact, in their skinny jeans, leather jackets, and vintage T-shirts, they look almost like the prototypical non-athlete. And before our interview, they step outside for a smoke. Still, the group's vital, stirring, and impressive; I wasn't there with her, but Julie's friends tell me she lost her mind at their show. Recently, Auerbach produced an amazing album for Dr. John, and Carney did a record for The Sheepdogs, the throwback Canadian rock band that wound up on the cover of *Rolling Stone*. They're not too cool to recommend a few tunes.

"Look at me. Clearly I'm not running anywhere, but I would definitely recommend listening to The Clash," Carney says.

"I'd say The Johnny Burnette Trio," says Auerbach. "You need something with a beat, something that's dance-y, and with great guitars." Johnny Burnette sings "Train Kept a Rollin'," which Aerosmith covers, and "You're Sixteen," which Paul McCartney sang with Ringo Starr on his album after The Beatles broke up. Ringo's record hit number one in 1974.

"I like The Cramps, The Cars—I bet you can run to anything that's just good music," says Carney, mentioning two groups that spent time in his home state, Ohio. The Cars are famous for "You Might Think" and "Good Times Roll," but I love, love, love "Just What I Needed," while The Cramps, part of the original CBGB movement, make punkish surf rock, best exemplified on songs like "Bikini Girls with Machine Guns" and "Tear It Up," a piece of punk rock perfection.

"I'm not going to run," continues Carney, "but if I was, I'd recommend any of the Sun Records bands." Started in 1952 by Sam Phillips in Memphis, Sun Record bands include Elvis Presley, Jerry Lee Lewis, Roy Orbison, and Johnny Cash.

AND NOW a few words about methodology, starring Katy Perry...

If you wonder how I got this list of running songs, the answer is by hook and by crook. Most of them came during an interview when the musician had something to promote. After speaking with whomever for my time allotted, a publicist would signal when I had time for one last question. This is when I would ask the artist to recommend a few running tunes.

In the case of Katy Perry, security was tighter than usual, and I wasn't even allotted the industry standard, twenty minutes of interview time. I was granted just three magic questions. What's more, the interview was conducted at Sears, where Perry was launching her perfume. Each of my questions had to pertain to her fragrance, which is called Purr (the new one's Meow!). I can't remember exactly how I started, but it's safe to assume it pertained to her smell.

For my last question, I inhaled. "Katy, if you were wearing your perfume," I said, "and running, what songs would you want to listen to, what songs could you recommend?"

"I love Rihanna," she said. "She has her own fragrance. And Rebecca Black, who sings "Friday"; the emotion is cuteness overall. A nice kind of lightness that goes well with my sense of humor."

There was a pause then, and the line behind me, which included television cameras and Sears security, began to press. I pressed back: "How about one more pick, Katy? And how about recommending one of your own tunes? You're wearing your perfume, about to go running, what song of your own would you play?"

"I guess for me, my song? 'Hummingbird Heartbeat' is a good one. It's fast, has a lot of double-entendres. I guess it's the one most like my perfume."

(Note: "Hummingbird Heartbeat" is 120 beats per minute. It is a good running song!)

21

WE NEED TO
TALK ABOUT
CORE STRENGTH

THE TRAINING: Attention to Detail

WEEK 42: Do one 8K (5-mile) easy run, one long run of 13K (8.1 miles), and one day of either hills or speed work, whichever you prefer. (For a good speed workout, try running 600 meters (650 yards) 8 times with a 2-minute light jog in between. The goal is to run the eighth interval as fast as the first. Hill runs, meanwhile, are what you'd expect: find a hill and run up and down it 6 or 8 times.)

WEEK 43: Run an easy 8K twice, and do one long run of 19K (11.8 miles). If you feel tired, sore, or overwhelmed, walk where you have to. Remember to bring bus fare and water.

THE SOUNDTRACK: Young Jeezy

THE FINISH LINE: The marathon, now just about 11 weeks away.

THE QUADRICEPS, abdomen, obliques, and glutes are your core muscles and, as you keep piling on mileage, they'll strengthen you and protect you from injury. Every new athlete's gung-ho to get out, buy sneakers, and start running; we want to break previous records and keep going farther and faster and we want to get there—get to our marathon—in the shortest possible time. We race when we're racing, and we race to get to the race. That's my basic mindset, and it seems to be the mantra of every runner, except, of course, Ed Whitlock, that I've ever met.

The thing is, most runners—Whitlock and myself included—have been injured, and this is why we need to build up our quadriceps, abdomen, obliques, and glutes (the muscles surrounding the torso) because they strengthen connective tissue, increase the durability of ligaments and joints, promote balance, and help stabilize the spine. Crashing, literally, your foot into the ground while you run, is a shock to your system. It's a collision. Core exercises help absorb the load.

"It's incredible how stupid you runners are; you do everything backwards," says Deirdre Casey, a competitive age group triathlete and Ironman finisher with platinum hair and a nose ring, who looks a little like Brigitte Nielsen, circa the second *Beverly Hills Cop.* "To be a good runner, you have to engage all your muscles, but you stupid runners—you just don't have the discipline to work on your core."

So, OK, I admit it: I don't always do my stupid core exercises, like lying face down on the floor and lifting myself up with my forearms and toes, which is called The Plank. This exercise also works the legs and shoulders, and Casey says if I just did this three times every night and every morning, perhaps five times for thirty seconds a rep, and switched between my left and right side to improve coordination, in two months, I'd be able to run my 3:05 in Boston. She says I'd recover faster after workouts, and I wouldn't have a knife stuck in my knee when I don't give myself enough time to recover between runs.

"You're only as strong as the weakest link in your body,"

Casey says, as she leads me through a series of exercises at a gym where Gordon Lightfoot pumps iron. The thing is, at Lightfoot's gym, Casey and I don't touch the machines. She tells me that not only are core exercises quick and essential but they can all be done at your house, in twenty minutes, with no equipment, for free.

"There are twenty-five variations of The Plank," says Casey, who's generally wearing leather pants when she's not wearing gym shorts, "but if you just lie on your stomach and lift your hands and feet and then switch to your side and lift your arm and leg—then switch sides and rotate once more through the cycle—it would be all the strength training you need for the marathon." It's best to do The Plank every day during your training, but it's essential to do it at least a few times a week. It's fine to Plank before going out on a short run but not before attempting 19K (11.8 miles)—your core gets worked out enough when you run that far. These next few weeks are going to be hard. Not only are you attempting to reach 19K, but you're also strongly encouraged to mix in alternating weeks of speed work and hills. With the marathon eleven weeks away, and your target for the long run 30K (18.6 miles), it's time to baby-proof your body.

RUNNERS WHO wore shoes made on waffle irons used to get in shape for running by running, and these guys drank G&Ts and ate nachos, cheeseburgers, and ice cream. Old school, they're called. Meanwhile, when Matt Loiselle tries to cut down his marathon time—it makes him angry that Jerome Drayton's Canadian marathon record of 2:10:09 still holds after almost forty years—he exercises his core. "It's more about fighting off injuries than getting a six-pack or huge muscles," says Loiselle, who was eighth with a 2:16:01 at the race in Toronto where Ed Whitlock was 296th.

We run together sometimes, Matt and I, and sometimes we go out afterward for Portuguese chicken and beer. One day he cycled me through the workout he does for his core. He keeps a boom box and a giant medicine ball on a tumbling mat in his garage, and following his afternoon shakeout run, an easy 8K (5 miles) after a morning of speed work, he kicks his legs up on top of the ball and lifts his hips up and down. He does this and also sits on the ground with a resistance band around his feet and leans his torso front and back, every day. "There are so many stupid small things with running that no one wants to do, but they're important," he says. "Even though they're annoying, they work."

All movement originates from the core: whether it's crawling, swimming, dancing, or running the marathon. These muscles help with balance; stabilize your body and it will generate the power you need in the marathon's last few kilometers when you're burning glycogen, having an anaerobic workout, losing all semblance of form, and, quite simply, holding on for dear life.

"Two thousand five, Lake Placid, when I won my first Ironman, I had nothing left in my legs. My core took me across the finish line," says Casey, back in our fancy gym in Toronto. Casey's won the women's master's division at Ironman events—which is beating the field of over-forty-year-olds—five times. "There's so many ways to become a better runner by doing a few simple exercises that help the body respond to the demands of endurance running. It boggles the mind that runners won't put in the time."

I'VE BEEN offered the chance to go to Jerusalem to run the marathon. I was going to use the Around the Bay 30K Road Race in Hamilton in March as a warm-up to Boston (if you're racing for a personal best, try a shorter race as a training run to break up your workouts and test your speed). So the plan for Jerusalem, after making certain that I don't have to pay for my airfare, is to go slow for the first 30K, then hit my race pace (4:23 per kilometer) during the final stretch. I've run three marathons, so I'm not afraid of the distance—but my goal in Boston is 3:05. I worry about speed.

The program I've written is the simplest one for completing your marathon. The program I follow is hell-bent on getting me across the finish line in Boston in 3:05: every Saturday, I do speed work or hills, and I run 20K (12.8 miles) on Tuesday and Thursday with Ben. On one of those runs, we do drills. This week, I ran my half-marathon pace five times for fifteen minutes (4:16 per kilometer). Next week, I'll do twelve out of my 20K at my marathon pace. I also run an easy 10K (6 miles) every Friday afternoon. It's convenient marathon training when three days a week you work from home and, on the other two, you're running into the office while helping your boss bring down his finishing time. I honestly don't know how people make the time for all this when they have to go into an office. Most of you probably already have a stronger core than I do.

I'VE MADE Esme laugh with my core exercises; they make me look like a cartoon. One is putting your socks on standing up and another is brushing your teeth on one leg. Running tests balance and coordination. And balance and coordination fall apart when you're beat. By working your core, you strengthen your center. It's like being glad during a hurricane that you installed sturdy beams in your home. Remember: we run on one foot; we're hoppers. When you do The Plank to the left and the right, you're isolating each side of your body. Seventeen kilometers (10.5 miles) into a 19K long run, you don't get the benefit of using both feet. You're only as strong as your weakest muscle, Deirdre Casey said. Core exercises strengthen the whole chain—all of which gets used, to its fullest, in the marathon. Here are three more core exercises she recommends.

How Stupid Runners Should Work on Their Core: A Wake-up Call, by Deirdre Casey

1. Hip hikes: Standing up, use your gluteal muscles (the muscles in your ass) to raise and lower your legs. Lift your leg straight out in front of you and try to get it parallel to the floor. Or bring your leg back behind you, but that's tougher. Try it both ways, on both sides, and do this ten or twelve times in sets of three.
2. Strides: Walk across your living room, exaggerating the motion so you reach all the way up to your full height and then all the way down to the ground on each leg. Lift your leg high and feel the flex in your abs.
3. Knee tucks: Sit against the wall with your hands on the ground and lift one knee to your chest, then the other. Repeat for three sets, ten or twelve times.

"The key thing about core strength for a runner is that you're trying to strengthen all of the muscles that will benefit all of your actions on one leg," says Dr. Kimitake Soto, an assistant professor in the Department of Kinesiology, Leisure, and Sport Sciences at East Tennessee State University. A lecturer in sports biomechanics, Soto says that none of the core muscle exercises are about quantity as much as they're about form. It doesn't matter how many you're doing; what matters is that you do them without twisting around.

Injuries occur when stronger muscles have to compensate for weaker ones. One way or the other, our bodies will keep us moving forward. Just as you can do the job of an inept co-worker for a while, eventually the strain will show on your own performance. You can only carry the load for so long. "Muscles don't work in isolation—all of our movements exist in a chain," says Dr. Soto, adding that weak hamstrings force the quads to compensate, which ends up pulling down the pelvis and hurting the back. "All of these things, little compensations, little erratic movements, little irregularities in the muscle chain—they're not a big deal in a 5K, but they can mean injury in a marathon."

To run 16K (10 miles) one week and 19K the next, you need to keep pounding the core. Deirdre Casey says that our bodies have four gears of core activation and that she always tries to stay engaged in at least gear number two (on a scale of one to four, where four is the highest). This makes sense. Train for your marathon beyond when you're running. When you're at your desk, sit up straight. And walk around every hour or so. Also, before you pick up your groceries, your baby, your laundry, your anything, tighten your abs. A lot of running injuries begin when we're not wearing sneakers. Eric Gillis, our friend who beat the Olympic qualifying time by one second, recently had trouble with his IT band, that strip of tissue that connects the hip to the lower leg. The reason? His kid had just started a new preschool, and Gillis was spending too much time in his car taking her there. Because he was sitting so often, and not engaging his core muscles, Gillis was tightening his hip flexors and the muscles in his back. The injury played itself out in his IT band: Canada's two-time Olympic runner was nearly done in by his carpool.

"There's no way to overestimate how important the core is to a runner," says Ron O'Hare, a physiotherapist who works with Gillis and changed the 2:11 marathon runner's workouts to include hip swings (lying on your side and moving your leg back and forth) and butterfly stretches (sitting on the floor with your back straight, the soles of your feet together making a diamond, and your elbows pushing down on your knees for ten seconds). Gillis took O'Hare's advice. And ran the marathon in the Olympics.

"It's great to get out there and eat up the miles, and enthusiasm and guts in a runner is key, but you have to bear in mind the everyday small stuff," O'Hare says. "Otherwise, it'll bite you in the ass."

THE SOUNDTRACK: Young Jeezy
The problem with interviewing rappers is that most of the very best ones smoke a lot of weed. It can be hard to speak with them, especially over the phone, and even harder to get them to keep an appointment. Once I waited seven hours for Snoop Dogg, and I swear to God I was supposed to interview Nicki Minaj forty-two separate times. That's why Young Jeezy was so surprising. Jeezy, born in Atlanta and a frequent collaborator of Kanye West and Jay-Z, called right on time and spoke candidly about Trayvon Martin, George Zimmerman, and that horrible shooting in Florida, plus what Obama's reelection means to his kids.

I asked him to rank himself as a performer: "There's Michael Jackson, and there's me," says Jeezy, and I like that; that's how you should feel when you race.

When pressed to recommend running songs, Young Jeezy confessed that he doesn't run. So I asked him two different questions: Before you're about to get onstage and compete against the ghost of Michael Jackson, what do you listen to? And what makes you feel good?

"When I'm sitting around drinking and smoking and getting ready to kill onstage in Canada, Norway, or London? If I'm not listening to Snoop Dogg or 2Pac or old Cash Money, then I'll listen to a little bit of Weezy [Lil Wayne], but there's definitely a lot of 'Pac in there." Jeezy said that 2Pac's *All Eyez on Me* is his favorite record when "everything's copasetic," but when he needs a burst of energy, he plays 2Pac's 1996 album *The Don Killuminati: The 7-Day Theory.** "I start that shit at number one and ride it out to number twelve, feel me?" asks Jeezy. "No one's ever done it like 2Pac, and Pac's never done it more passionately, with more fire, than he does on this shit right here."

* The most famous track on *The Don Killuminati* is "Hail Mary," which took thirty minutes to record and will live forever. When 2Pac appeared as a hologram at the Coachella Valley Music and Arts Festival in 2012, it was "Hail Mary" he screamed.

22

LESSONS FROM
THE FRINGE

THE TRAINING: Introducing Workout Number Four

WEEK 44: Run 8K (5 miles), do 1 run of speed work or hills, try 35 minutes on the rowing machine (or swim or bike instead), and go for a beautiful 14K (18.7-mile) long run.

WEEK 45: Stick with your 8K run and 35 minutes of rowing, biking, or swimming; try another 8 or 10K (5 to 6 miles), running lightly; and do a 24K (14.9-mile) long run, which seems like a lot but is only 3K (1.9 miles) more than the half-marathon.

THE SOUNDTRACK: Pearl Jam

THE FINISH LINE: The marathon, now just 9 weeks away!

SCOTT JUREK is an American ultramarathon runner from Seattle who set a record that sounds a little like torture: on a mile-long loop, he covered the greatest distance in history of any American runner over a twenty-four-hour period. For every second of May 12, 2011, he ran in circles, and even though he's an experienced madman—twice he won the

Badwater Ultramarathon, a 135-mile (217-kilometer) race in California's Death Valley—something about the circles and the course, the amount of time spent on his feet, and the lack of distractions, made this challenge a particular nightmare.

"The first eight hours weren't too bad. Obviously, they got to be monotonous, going around in circles, but I got into a rhythm and stayed within my race," he says. "At about twelve hours, though, things started changing. I began to think, boy, this is going to be a long night." You may feel something similar when you embark on next week's ambitious long run—24K (14.9 miles). You can do it. It's just 5K (3 miles), four times, with a little under one more 5K thrown in. But it's longer than the island of Manhattan and probably farther than you've ever been running before. It's normal to think, like Scott Jurek, boy, this is going to be a long day. Nobody runs the marathon and thinks, ah, just a lovely walk in the park.

First, we're doing 14K (8.7 miles) as a long run, to allow a little rest from last week, mixed, of course, with an easy run of 8K (5 miles), some speed work, and thirty-five minutes on the rowing machine (or on the bike or in the pool). Next week, do 8K twice—we need to build up the mileage—and also thirty-five minutes of cross-training, something to keep building strength in your core. But the big thing right now is your long run: 24K is a distance vast enough to cross Chicago almost twice. Don't lose track of the fact that what you're doing is difficult. If you don't find it difficult, frankly, you're wrong.

DOES YOUR schedule demand that you skip a run this week? That's fine, but don't back out on your long run. And if you feel a nagging sense of angst or frustration, that's normal. I feel it. And so do Ryan Hall and Deena Kastor, Kathrine Switzer and Wesley Korir. Everyone feels it. And you can be damned sure that, running around in circles for twenty-four hours, Scott Jurek felt exactly the same thing. "Fear of failure, creeping doubt, this nagging sense of hopelessness—I'm just like everybody else out there running; these thoughts begin to creep in," says Jurek, who adds that part of being a successful endurance runner is developing the mental strength to block out these thoughts when they start to invade. Every run has its stages. The trick is to power through the bad stages and have faith that they won't last. For Scott Jurek, after running for sixteen hours, very appropriately, he began to go nuts.

"I thought I was losing my mind," he tells me. "I felt like I can't do this anymore. I was at a real low point, but then I began listening to music, everything from Rage Against the Machine to hip hop, and then, with seven hours to go, I started focusing," says Jurek, who would go on to run 266.7 kilometers (165.7 miles) in twenty-four hours, the equivalent of almost six-and-a-half marathons, doing the entire thing around a godforsaken one-mile track. "I got out of my funk and started finding small goals to bring me back into the present and focused on my technique and little challenges—if I could just make it around that stupid loop one more time," he says. "It was probably the most challenging mental obstacle I've ever competed in, but the emotions—the effort it required—is really no different than what anyone else feels who's attempting a race."

The beauty of running is how specific the task is. There is only one thing you have to do: go forward. And like Jurek, who gets off on doing the inconceivable, you too will just need to focus, stay positive, and keep moving ahead. Every step you take is one more step closer toward your final destination. Organization is the key to both training and reaching the finish line: knowing what your pace should be, what you need for your journey, and what you should do to be properly prepared.

Whether it's running around in circles for twenty-four hours or getting your long run up to 24K, running gives you the opportunity to experiment with your boundaries. And even if you fail, you tried. Say you go out for 19K and only do twelve. So what? You just ran 12K (7.4 miles)! How much better is that than eating another corned beef sandwich and two stacks of Pringles? And what's more, you're probably already reaping the benefits of your endeavor, whether that's losing a few pounds, sleeping better, or staying home on a couple more Friday nights. Remember, it doesn't matter how long it takes you to finish your marathon. What matters is that you get out there and try.

Thirteen million people finished some kind of race last year in the U.S. Only 500,000 of them ran the marathon. And here you are, going for it. Plus, odds are, after you do it once, you'll do it again. Who wants to learn how to fly a jet plane and then only go up in the air once? Just think of this marathon as a warm-up, literally, a test run. It's not the last episode of *Dexter*. It's not even prom: there's no one you need to impress.

"In fact, if you have to prove something to someone else, that's flawed logic. There's no greater person to prove something to than yourself. Why are you trying to impress anybody?" asks Kelly Gneiting, father of five who lives in Fort Defiance, Arizona, and set a world record at the LA Marathon in 2011: he weighed four hundred pounds at the start and had lost nearly four pounds by the time he finished in 9:48:52, becoming the heaviest marathon finisher of all time. Gneiting is a truck driver and American sumo wrestler, whose sport demands three- or four-second bursts of power and speed. Curious about the discipline of the marathon—could he actually do something for so long?—he mulled over the idea until one day, while refueling his semi in Columbus, Montana, Gneiting reached a decision: come hell or high water, he was running the marathon. The actual race, however, was another story.

"It's like overall leprosy of your inner organs," says Gneiting, who ran for so long on that wet morning in Los Angeles that he first felt blisters on his feet forming and then felt them burst. "It was just Wall after Wall after Wall to break through, but I began to think of the end as Christmas morning. Just a little bit further, and I could celebrate with my wife of eighteen years and my kids."

Rest assured, your marathon's going to be nothing like running 42.2K over nine hours at four hundred pounds. But there will probably be moments out there when you'll be able to relate to Gneiting's vibe. Come to think of it, you've already probably felt "overall leprosy of your inner organs" on long training runs or in your 10K race or even just out on a routine Sunday morning when you either ate badly or dressed wrong or desperately needed to use a bathroom you couldn't find. Every runner's been there. The important thing is how you get through it. Maybe you need to hydrate better, shun lactose, swap mittens for gloves, or remember to wear sunglasses when running on a buggy path. For Gneiting, it turns out the adage about what doesn't kill you was true.

"When I crossed the finish line, it was raining and, man, right before, maybe ten or twenty yards, I started crying a little bit," he says. "I didn't want anyone to see me, and then when I crossed, just after, I collapsed. I looked at the sky, looked at everybody, and said 'Thank You,' then sat down. I'd accomplished my goal."

DR. JOEL FISH is the director of the Center for Sport Psychology in Philadelphia and works with the Phillies, 76ers, and Flyers. Philadelphia fans are notoriously honest—they once booed a shoddy Santa Claus—and athletes competing in that city have a heavy cross to bear. But whether you're Allen Iverson, Mike Schmidt, or my mother-in-law getting ready for her first 5K, the same negative thoughts can become a distraction. "The most common mental block is fear of failure, but what also holds us back is perfectionism: I'm not going to try to do this because there's no way I can do it well," says Dr. Fish, who also works with the U.S. women's national soccer team. "For me, sports psychology is about coming up with a good mental plan to incorporate along with the technical game plan an athlete follows to reach a performance goal."

Dr. Fish recommends a bunch of different ways to prepare for your race. The first, and perhaps most popular, is to incorporate positive self-talk and good mental imagery. Stop saying how difficult the race will be and instead focus on the finish line. You've run 5K; you've run 10 K; you've done the half-marathon. Why should the marathon be any different? And many people who do this are just like you. The night before the race, instead of worrying about how cold it will be or how many training runs you skipped, think about what you're going to eat after the run. Picture yourself having brunch with your friends, wearing a medal around your neck, drinking a Guinness—having completed something most people are too afraid to try.

"It's all about reframing experiences and seeing them in a different way: this is something we want and are actively seeking. Not a crisis, it's an opportunity," says Dr. Fish. "Enjoy it. Something like running the marathon is a novel, authentic experience; make it a memory that you want to last. It's yours. Make the most of it, and do it for yourself." Running isn't something that you should do. It's something you *choose* to do. There's a difference between taking marching orders and calling your own shots.

This is just like how Scott Jurek talks about his vegan diet. I asked him what was hardest to give up, and he told me that he didn't give up anything. He gained something—a healthier style of eating and a better way of life. "I'm not denying myself anything," he says. "For me, being vegan isn't a diet of deprivation; it's a diet of integration. It seems hard, but once you get into it, it doesn't have to be this chore. It's a journey. It's fun."

IN JERUSALEM, the marathon course is unbelievably challenging—all hills and tight turns and mountains coming one after the other, like hiccups. There I meet a woman named Jennifer Scroggins from Northern Kentucky who works for a newspaper in Ohio and makes a mistake that I pray you won't. She got to the starting line of her half-marathon and pounded forward—up Ammunition Hill, through the extraordinarily tight Armenian Quarter, and down and around both the German and Greek Colonies. When it started to hail, Scroggins didn't quit—even though she'd gotten a stomach bug on her first night in Israel.

"I'm such a bad runner it's not even funny," she told me, and then added that she doesn't even like running, has no interest in speed work, and just sort of "magically hoped to wake up being faster one day. I'm actually not entirely certain what I want to get out of running," she said. "Maybe that's what my problem is." It was such a revelation to me when she told me her story because I was blown away by how well she ran. This was a brutal course in tough conditions, she was under the weather, and she triumphed—yet she was still bummed out after her race.

It's important that you set reasonable expectations. Maybe you want to finish. Or maybe you want to run without walking. Perhaps you're trying to come in at some arbitrary time.

Doesn't matter. The point is: don't set yourself up for disappointment. If you haven't trained, don't expect to run like Scott Jurek; and if you're running for fun, don't forget that at the finish line. The problem with having timed races is that everyone receives a score. It sucks being scored, and it subverts the best part of running—being healthy, getting in shape, having a goal, being a good parent, doing anything other than developing blisters on your hands from overusing your television's remote control. And race organizers and health promoters know this, which is why they're introducing color runs, zombie runs, obstacle courses, dance parties, and other noncompetitive events. If things are getting too heavy, this can be a good way to put the fun back into running and involve other members of your support community who wouldn't otherwise join you. I make the mistake too often of choking the life out of things. Don't do that to your hobby.

In Jerusalem, I ran my best marathon and had my worst finishing time. In Toronto, I scored 3:08:40; in Israel, I hit 3:32:21. But even though I ran through hail, wind, and pretty much everything other than boils and frogs, I never felt like I wanted to charge an Israeli soldier and have her put me out of my misery. There was no point in that race where I wasn't smiling, and when I turned on my jets at 30K (18.6 miles), it felt good. I wasn't green.

Nine weeks out from your marathon, answer some questions. Do you want to push yourself to the breaking point and run as fast as humanly possible, until you can't move your legs or control your bowels? Or do you want to run comfortably, eat lunch with your children afterward, and show off your race shirt? Either of these goals is acceptable, but the trick to enjoying your race and, in turn, to enjoying running is to acknowledge what you're setting out to do and what you're doing it for. That way, you may even do it again.

THE SOUNDTRACK: Pearl Jam

If I were held over a flaming cauldron, I'd say Pearl Jam's my favorite group. Julie's friend saw their concert and described seeing a stadium of middle-aged men in short pants having a religious experience. I was at that concert in short pants. And I had that kind of experience. Let's just say I'm glad Julie was at home with baby Es. Anyway, when I got a chance to interview the band, I spoke with every member except Eddie Vedder, the singer, who's not unlike Bono or Bruce Springsteen. I waited in the hotel room, and when the band arrived, we had a terrific discussion. Then I asked, "What's it feel like to have to do these interviews for Eddie, who won't talk to the press?" Stone Gossard, who plays guitar, said: "Oh, he'll do them. He just wouldn't do one with you."

Matt Cameron, the band's drummer, is actually a pretty serious runner, but he doesn't run with music. "It takes you out of your body," he says. "Plus, sometimes when you run in the city, it's a little dangerous. Sometimes a car will come up on your backside."

I kind of thought Pearl Jam might not give me any running tunes. But there's a reason they're my favorite rock band. Gossard spoke up.

Motörhead, *Ace of Spades*: "Matt's really the band's runner, but I still highly recommend cranking Motörhead. *Ace of Spades*—it's hard to get harder than that."

This prompted Jeff Ament, the bassist, to chime in:

Led Zeppelin, "Achilles Last Stand": "This is one of the great skate songs. It should also probably get you where you want to get to on a run."

23

AN OLIVE BRANCH
TO THE SLACKERS

THE TRAINING: Your Last Session of Four Workouts a Week

WEEK 46: Stick with 8K (5 miles) twice this week, mix in speed work or hills, and try a recovery run of 16K (10 miles).

WEEK 47: Run 8K easy, twice; spend 35 minutes rowing (or swimming or cycling); and do a long run of 27K (16.7 miles). Walk where you have to and keep track of how long it takes: the goal is to finish, but it helps to have an idea of your average time per kilometer (or mile, of course).

THE TRAINING for Slackers:

WEEK 46 (Week 1): Get out 3 times this week for 9K (5.6 miles) each session and walk as need be, perhaps for 1 minute every other kilometer.

WEEK 47 (Week 2): Stick with 9K twice, but then add a long run—try 15K (9.3 miles).

WEEK 48 (Week 3): If you can handle 15K, drop your two 9Ks to seven (4.3 miles), and shoot for an 18K (11.1-mile) long run. This will get you back in the game again with a long run goal of 30K (18.6 miles).

THE SOUNDTRACK: Norah Jones, plus Carrie Underwood on Mötley Crüe

THE FINISH LINE: The marathon, now just about 7 weeks away.

WE'RE BUILDING up to 27K (16.7 miles) but, for those who have been keeping up with the training, first we're going back down a little to allow for recovery after last week's long run. This week, keep momentum up with a couple of 8K (5-mile) runs and some speed work (perhaps four or five one-mile repeats in which the last mile is as fast as the first one) or hills. The long run is only at 16K (10 miles)—and I use the word "only" respectfully, but by now, hopefully, you've run that a bunch—because you'll need fresh legs for next week's challenge. As you approach 27K, nearly seventeen miles, make sure you bring some water if you're running in the heat. Waistbelts and hydration packs now work so seamlessly you'll almost forget you're wearing them. There's no exact formula for drinking; the latest from the International Marathon Medical Directors Association is to drink when you get thirsty. (It took an entire association to come up with that.) I generally take some water every 5K (3 miles), and if it's really sunny, Julie makes me wear a hat.

Regardless, take precautions. I realize you may have signed up for the marathon in a flourish of enthusiasm or New Year's Day guilt and followed this training, in earnest, for a bit. Now, however, the marathon's approaching and those Asics you bought may be gathering dust like my grandmother's painting of an old lady giving an egg to a young man that I borrowed from Aunt Linda, which I really wanted at the time. It's OK. There is hope.

"You can't make up for lost time, but you can maximize seven weeks," says Reid Coolsaet, who shares a dirty little secret about his own training. In 2009, he ran his first marathon after preparing for less than two months. "I'd broken my foot and then returned to running and had this idea in my head to run the marathon," says Coolsaet, adding that six intense weeks of training does have its advantages. When training a year for something, your energy ebbs and flows like your attention span. But when you zoom in on a goal intensely for a few hot weeks—like cramming for a test or working around the clock to make a deadline—the intensity can turn a negative into a strength.

"It's exciting, a bit of a gamble, a bit of a risk—like playing the lottery—and my training became thrilling. I wanted to do this, but I didn't know what to expect," Coolsaet says. "I had no idea what it was going to feel like, but for those six weeks, I thought about it every day and trained as hard as I could."

For the people who've been keeping up, this is halftime—a nice minute to take stock before digging in. Good luck on your 27K. Don't forget to air dry your race shirt.

The rest of you slackers—those exhibiting the same tendencies I showed back in math class, when at first I didn't do the work because I couldn't be bothered and then because I didn't have a clue how to do it—welcome to marathon running. It's done by spending lots of time running around. If you've run the half, you can get to the marathon in seven weeks if you haven't been keeping up with the program. But you've got to start running right now. No more feeling apathetic and hopeless; that's finished. It's a new day, so during Week 46 (or whatever week it is now for you—might as well start counting it as Week 1), go slow, slow, slow and just get yourself reacquainted with the sport. Try to get out three times this week, but don't push. Don't worry about speed or even distance, though if you're hitting between 7 and 9K (4.3 and 5.6 miles), great. We're just reintroducing you to all this running stuff. You liked it once; let's get back into it again. Sign up for a marathon.

If you hit 9K three times during your reorientation, the following week, Week 2, introduce the long run. You really don't want to move up week by week by more than 3K (1.9 miles), but, for starters, see where you're at. Tuck cab money or bus fare into your pocket and try a 15K (9.3-mile) long run. If you've done the half, you should have the muscle memory for endurance running. Go slowly, above everything, and walk where you need to. The week after that, Week 3, after hitting a 15K long run, drop your 9Ks to seven, do them twice, rest, and move your long run to 18K (11.1 miles). With a month to go until the marathon, this distance will get you within striking distance of completing 42K (26 miles).

These numbers don't have to be exact. The point is to build your mileage without burning out. Everyone's starting from somewhere different, but use those distances to ballpark your progress. Write everything down and engage your core. Flex your stomach muscles and use the stairs. Substitute baby carrots for chips. If you're excited, work in a day of cross-training, perhaps thirty minutes on a rowing machine, or else swim or ride a bike. Skip the Jägermeister, cut out the Johnnies, but remain realistic: there's nothing quite like the marathon.

"The marathon's a quantum leap from the half-marathon; it hurts like nothing else," says Ralph Vernacchia, adding that you can slack off on your training and finish the half-marathon, but that the marathon knocks out the unprepared. "Nothing worse than seeing someone who hasn't trained try to run the marathon. It's like sending a guy who can't surf into Waikiki with a board and a prayer."

According to Vernacchia, there are a couple of ways to avoid being that poor surfer. First off, run part of the actual marathon course in training, cutting it into two sections. This way, you'll know what to expect and there'll be no surprises. Second, Vernacchia, like John Stanton, Mickey Hall, and the best Kenyan coaches, believes the way to the marathon is through the weekly long run, so if you're going to skip something (and you probably are), don't skip that. Try to increase your long run distance by 3K (1.9 miles) each week. Generally, if you can run thirteen, you can run sixteen, and if you can run sixteen, you can run nineteen. Once you hit nineteen, you begin to approach the magic number of thirty. Once you're there—goes Vernacchia's theory, anyway—you can run 42.2.

"If you can do seventeen miles two weeks before your race, you'll be fine—though you wouldn't really be racing. It's more like a survival jog," says Vernacchia, adding that there's a difference between "getting through" your marathon and enjoying it. The better prepared you are, the more fun you'll have. However, there's one essential point of race-day preparedness, which affects everyone from Olympians on down: no matter how strong you feel in the beginning, do not burn yourself out at the start. "The difference between completing the marathon and dropping out is your pace," he says, adding that during your training runs it's imperative that you monitor your time. You need to know about how long it takes you to run a kilometer (or a mile) so that you can figure out how much time to expect your entire marathon might be. It's all about knowing what to plan for. And so, on your long run, jot down your total time and also try to practice running consistently at one speed. Going one speed for your entire marathon is easier than speeding up and slowing down across 26.2 miles.

On race day, at the starting line, you'll feel nervous and excited. But talk to the other people around you. Find someone who looks more experienced at racing than you. If you approach someone who seems trustworthy, and shares your finishing goal, stick to that person during the race. Let him or her set the pace and don't think about anything, but be cautious. Because even if you knock out 30K (18.6 miles) in training, that last 12K (7.4 miles) is where the marathon begins. Don't get me wrong, you can do this—but not if you go too fast, too soon.

"A marathon's about the equal distribution of energy and resources over an extended period of time," says Vernacchia. "You don't wake up one morning and say you're going to Okinawa: you need a map, you need some hustle, and you need a plan."

THE OTHER THING you need, especially if you've been slacking, is good food and rest. Jason Riley is the director of sports performance at The Performance Compound in Tampa, Florida, and he made his name keeping Derek Jeter immortal. According to Riley, when you're seven weeks away from the marathon, it's no different from a Yankee being a month away from the start of the season—everything can use a tweak. "I have my guys keep a food log and write down whatever goes into their mouth, and not only what they eat or drink, but how much," says Riley, who also trains the Phillies' Ryan Howard and tennis player Maria Sharapova.

With the marathon quickly approaching, and training (for some of us) to this point being less than superb, it's important to grab hold of every advantage. And so in addition to avoiding the obvious stuff like malt liquor, cronuts, and bacon and goat sandwiches, Riley also says fried foods, sugar, and processed food stuffs, things like Froot Loops and Cheez-Its, can become a hindrance to recuperating after a long run. "Marathon training is all about recovery, since you're constantly staking out new ground and you need to constantly be rebuilding your muscles. Stuff like soft drinks, cooking oils, and fatty cuts of red meat can give athletes an inflammatory response to the food," says Riley, who could've included dairy in his list, and emphasizes that you don't have to radically alter your eating— he wouldn't ask Shaq to become a vegetarian seven weeks out from opening night—but slight alterations could contribute to a general toning. (And when you're running four hours across twenty-six miles, you feel every last bite of goat sandwich you eat.)

"Fruits, vegetable, salads—things you can digest easily—are good," says Riley, to which I'll add swapping multigrain for white bread, salmon for steak, watermelon for ice cream, and gobbling mixed nuts as an in-front-of-the-television snack. Also, seven weeks away from my marathon? I completely abstain from booze.

"WHILE YOU TRAIN, visualize race scenarios and picture yourself crossing the finish line," says Kimberley Amirault-Ryan, head of the mental performance team of Canada's Olympic Committee. According to Amirault-Ryan, who also worked with the Rangers and the Knicks—and helped them refocus on sports after 9/11—it's important to break the last few weeks of your training down into manageable nuggets. Don't worry about what you haven't done, but get organized. Figure out when you're running each week and stick to those times.

"With seven weeks left to go, book your life around your training," says Amirault-Ryan, adding that this intense period of focus should be fun: You're alive! Even if it isn't fun, too bad—we don't want you backing out of a race. So take a deep breath, and get out those shoes. "Act yourself to a feeling. Don't wait for a sensation to overcome you—'Oh, I feel like a gazelle today, I'm going to run freely through the wild'—doesn't happen," she says. She also tells her Olympic athletes to keep perspective: running your first marathon might feel like attending the Oscars, but overanalysis can lead to paralysis. Chill out and enjoy the event; there will always be another race.

"Every day, just do the little things you can do that you have direct control over," she says. "If you've been slacking with your training till now, forget about it. It's not over. Besides, anything's better than sitting on the couch all day eating chips."

THE SOUNDTRACK: Norah Jones

The woman who introduced Julie and me had a boyfriend who played in a punk band. He was a great friend of mine, a Lower East Side Buddha, and when he and the woman who introduced Julie and me broke up, he had the blues and was housebound. All he did was listen to Norah Jones. I'm tempted to tell Norah Jones this—she's friendly and approachable and smaller than you'd think, and during our conversation she has a little schmear of hummus on her nose—but I feel tongue-tied.

"Where should we go? You want to do it in the bedroom?" she asks me, about our interview, I suppose, and I just stand there, thinking, God, this is such a great job.

When I ask her to recommend some running songs, she said, "Running? You mean jogging?" And after I said, "Kinda. It's just a little bit more intense," she gives me two songs she thought you might like (and I make a note to email my friend).

"Getting Up," Q-Tip: "That's a good jogging song. It's fun." Q-Tip, of course, is the leader of A Tribe Called Quest and without him, there's no Kanye West, Frank Ocean, or Drake. We've already established that beats-per-minute alone do not make a great running song, but the Tribe track "Keep it Rol-lin'" is, indeed, at that rhythm. (And if you like Q-Tip and want another recommendation, "Definition" by Mos Def and Talib Kweli as Black Star is at that same tempo. I'm sure Norah would approve.)

"Everybody Knows This Is Nowhere," Neil Young: "It's not the first Neil Young song I fell in love with, but it's a good one to run with. He says [singing]: *I gotta get away/from this day-to-day/running around.* I know that's not the kind of running that you're talking about, but I still think it's probably all right for jogging. It's got a good pep."

Bonus Cut: Carrie Underwood on Mötley Crüe
Carrie Underwood is in the *Guinness Book of World Records* for having the most No. 1 country hits of any female artist in the U.S. This is mindboggling, since she was only introduced to the world on *American Idol* in 2005. The daughter of a saw-mill worker, Underwood is married to a hockey player and is a fan of Aerosmith and Randy Travis. "I'm all about hard rock music when I work out," she tells me and then gives a run-down on her favorite CD.

"*Dr. Feelgood* by Mötley Crüe is my favorite running record, because the songs motivate me and make me hunker down," she says, mentioning that she covered "Home Sweet Home" on *American Idol* in 2009. "I want something that's loud, with drums and great vocals, and I can listen to any Möt-ley Crüe record, but *Dr. Feelgood* is what I keep coming back to. It's fun to rock, you know? It makes you forget how hard you're working."

24

LOVE IN THE TIME
OF SNEAKERS

THE TRAINING: The Dirty Thirty

WEEK 48: Run 8 to 10K (5 to 6 miles) at race pace, try speed work or hills, and do a recovery long run of 12K (7.4 miles).

WEEK 49: Stick with 2 runs of 8 to 10K each, super easy, rest, and eat carbohydrates, then blast your last long run: 30K (18.6 miles, walk wherever you need to).

THE SOUNDTRACK: Feist

THE FINISH LINE: The marathon, now just about 5 weeks away!

AS YOU CUT OUT alcohol and movie popcorn, get as religious about your training program as Will Smith and Tom Cruise, and insist on resting up every Saturday night for the next morning's long run, there's a chance that you'll wind up with something like a sneaker up your ass. Assure your loved ones, as we turn the screws ever tighter, that your marathon now is only five weeks away.

"Put away the dickhead," Julie says to me one magic morning, as the baby cries right around 3 a.m. How do I respond to her honestly, that I'm actually about to ramp up the dickhead, get even more anal about what I eat and when I sleep, what I'll do and won't do, as a year's worth of training is about to get tested at the Boston Marathon in a month?

FIVE WEEKS OUT from the marathon, we're going to keep ramping up the long run, but this is it—this is the last time. Take the long runs slowly. Fight through the pain and know it's a cycle, that the bad feelings won't last. Also, deep breaths help ward off cramps, and walking for a minute every thirty minutes might actually help you complete your 30K (18.6 miles) faster than if you try, and fail, to run the whole thing. Play Brian Wilson on your iPod, play Norah Jones, and whatever you do, don't give up.

At the same time, we're back down to three workouts. This week, on an 8 to 10K (5- to 6-mile) run, try doing the distance at the pace you plan on running your marathon. Take stock of how you're feeling, and if you feel strong, try this for speed: two 800s, two 600s, four 400s, and one 200-meter sprint. That'll wake you up in the morning.

Next week, your goal is to cross the 30K threshold. Forget about speed work and just twice run 8 or 10K easy, saving everything for your distance goal. Once you cross 30K, you can do forty-two. So after that, breathe easy. We'll keep running, but the most important thing you can do at that point is avoid overtraining injuries (and cars).

Meanwhile, you slackers, no smoking. How are you? You guys should've maxed out last week at 18K (11.1 miles) and so now rest a bit, and run 10K three times. Then, next week, do 7K (10.5 miles) twice and shoot for a 23K (14.2-mile) long run. It's not a perfect training distance, but it's more than the half-marathon. If your marathon is still at least three weeks away, try to get your long run up to 26K (16.2 miles) the week after next. Two weeks from the marathon, no more adding distance and no more running beyond 14K (8.7 miles).

EVERYTHING YOU do now is a race rehearsal: what you eat for dinner, what you have for breakfast, which shorts you wear, whether or not you wear sunglasses, compression socks, a hat. Do you take energy gels? Do you carry water? Do you know how you're getting to the race? Simulate in practice what you're going to do in your marathon. Begin formulating your strategy, and take a look at the course map or else run a bit of the actual route if there's time. If you're paying money to participate, it makes sense to get involved. Enjoy this time: think about how the days leading up to your vacation can be more fun than the actual trip (and that's when you're not running 26.2 miles). Want to allay errant nerves and nervous energy? Make a plan and edit it obsessively, then ease back and wait for your chance to shine.

"My job is to take hope out of the equation," says Dr. Trent Stellingwerff, head of innovation and research at the Canadian Sport Institute and physiologist to Canada's Olympic athletes, including his wife. "So many people go into a race without doing a true gut check. They might have a goal pace but have never come close to that time in training, and then they wonder why they start cramping or blow up in the marathon."

Every coach I've talked to repeats a variation of these same eight words: *don't pray for a miracle on race day.* According to Stellingwerff, the most important part of your training five weeks from race day is the specificity of your workouts. Concentrate on each lap of your speed days, and don't be afraid to push on the last kilometer of your 30K run. Train; don't go through the motions. Remember, if running is boring, you're doing it wrong. However, and this is an oxymoron and I'm sorry, also use caution—don't add distance to these training runs and don't get hurt. The long run should top off at 30K; there's no need to run any farther than that.

"People get nervous and they get excited and they give the whole game away before even getting to the starting line," Stellingwerff says. "I see this all the time in marathon runners—and not just in first-timers, but pros." When you're out on your 30K long run, use your imagination. Simulate the race. Where do you need to walk? During some of my training runs, I run slowly, but I push my race pace for three fifteen-minute intervals. That's a good exercise for running on tired legs, and I almost never run anymore without attempting at least some kind of drill. But some experts don't do any of these things. Ed Whitlock keeps his running much simpler. He runs every day for three hours at the same speed so that when he gets to a marathon starting line, it's just another Tuesday. He does the same thing every day.

"If you expect to run a five-hour marathon, I'm not saying to go out on a five-hour jog, but I strongly suggest doing something in training for five hours," Stellingwerff says, recommending combining a cross-training session with a long run to make up that time. "Psychologically, doing something for five hours is massive. Knock it off once first in practice. That way, when you get to the starting line, you aren't scared."

ON RACE DAY, you also don't want to be at war with the world. "If you frown, you tighten up. The best thing I can recommend is to smile," says Ron Hill, the winner of the 1970 Boston Marathon, who's run every day since December 20, 1964. He was sixth in the 1972 marathon at the Berlin Olympics, run only five days after eleven Israeli athletes and coaches were killed.

His best marathon time is 2:09:28, which was then a world record—he's the first person to break 2:10—and even though he ran on the day he broke his pelvis in a car crash, he says he's really no different than you.

"If you've kept up with your training, relax and let good feelings occupy the breadth of your mind," says Hill, whose advice is reminiscent of what I learned from Sam Cohen, founder of *Canadian Running*, whom I met in Jerusalem. On the night before race day, because he's thirsty but also to remind himself to stay loose, Cohen allows himself a few beers. "Running twenty-six miles is bloody hard, especially if you're setting out to break your previous record or finish a race of that distance for the first time," Hill says. "Don't put any additional burdens on yourself. In fact, your goal from about five weeks on should be how to best tuck those additional burdens away." It's very difficult to run when you're wound up so tightly that if you find another runner's watch on the path, you give it a swift kick into the woods.

I HAVE a plan I'm proud of for Boston. Since I can't find shorts with two zippered pockets—one for my iPod and one for my gels—I'm going to wear a shirt with a pocket, along with the zip-pocketed shorts I've worn each time I've raced. I've studied the course and updated my music (Pearl Jam! Feist! Dolly Parton!) for about thirty-five minutes' worth, which is all I want. I'll turn it on at 2:10, which should see me just past the Newton Fire Station, approaching 30K and, God willing, the finish line. I'll then tuck the iPod away and run the last 5 or 6K (3 miles) listening to the screaming of crazy New England.

Everyone prepares for race day in their own way. "I get focused on what I'm eating in the month leading up to the marathon. I start to think about not eating crap," says Lesley

Taylor, whose own training was derailed last month when she dropped out of the 30K Around the Bay race because she set out on a pace too fast. Taylor's run six marathons, twenty halfs, Around the Bay another six times, and three Ironmans. It doesn't matter. You can still blow up at any time. Next month, she's running the London Marathon. For now, her training's all about fine-tuning, eating and resting well, getting her confidence back.

"I have a 32K long run this weekend and then I begin my taper. I'm just hoping my ankle doesn't give me fits," she says, adding that she's attempting to give up alcohol and cookies but also trying not to get too obsessed. "I try not to change too much in the month before a marathon. There's temptation to experiment and get radical, but by now you should know yourself as a runner and accept that. At this point, you've already established how you will run."

ON MY thirty-seventh birthday, I woke up thinking there had got to be a pill to erase thirty-seven beers. On my thirty-eighth, I wake up and take a long walk with my mom. It's been a year since I started out on this quest to run Boston, and when my parents come to town to see Esme, I cook them dinner for the first time.

Esme's crawling, and Julie uses the Magic Bullet to moosh her veggies and I'm telling all this to Joan Rivers, explaining to her that I can't believe Julie and I, who are great at big romantic gestures but still battle too often about putting the peanut butter away, have this smiling bouncing little girl. I tell her that running's been helpful, that it keeps me regular, and she says that comedy does the same thing for her.

"Obviously I was in great distress when my husband died, but I never left the spotlight. I found it very comforting,"

Rivers says. Her husband committed suicide right after they launched their talk show in 1987, and she only stopped performing then out of respect to her daughter, Melissa, who couldn't understand her mom's yen to get back to work. Work provided Rivers with a refuge, a place where she understood what she had to do, and felt safe and in control. Running does the same thing for me, and hopefully it's etched its way into your bones.

"I understand people who go running on the day a tragedy happens or at times of great stress; it takes your mind off it," she says. "After Edgar killed himself—and I'm not afraid to use those words, because they're important; it's important not to push that under the rug—but after he did that, Melissa and I went away. She was a wreck, and you have to get your priorities straight, but I couldn't wait to get back out there. I got back on that horse as fast as I could."

When Ron Hill was at the Munich Olympics, chaos reigned. He couldn't get the image of those eleven athletes out of his head—until he started running. Like Gilbert Kiptoo running Vancouver after the death of his father, Hill finally found a sense of relief in the marathon. "I think all of the runners competing that day were quite happy indeed when we got past the starting line," says Hill, who was a favorite to win Munich but wound up a few places behind Frank Shorter, the American distance runner whose gold medal kicked off the first great running boom. "Running is something I hold sacred. I see it as a part of my person, and racing's just an expression of all that training. You shouldn't be nervous; you should feel thrilled."

One of my favorite running personalities is Thelma Wright, who ran in the 1972 and 1976 Olympics. She says that if you stopped training right now, it would be better for you than if you did too much. I find that comforting. "Why are you running?" Wright asks. "Is it social, physical, for your mental well-being? To run a successful marathon, you have to figure out what your goals are. Everyone has their own definition of what it would mean to win."

Running provides me with sanctuary; it's an escape and a challenge but also a place to think and relax. Keep that in mind with your training, especially this close to race day. Don't make the running a struggle; try to bury the dickhead, and fight to make running a refuge from all the other struggles you have.

THE SOUNDTRACK: Feist

Of the twenty-nine musicians we've featured, Feist is the only one I contacted specifically to provide running songs. It was at her concert that I came up with my half-marathon approach to footwear (wearing pink racing flats around Vegas and then switching into something a little more substantial for the race), and when I was left alone with Esme in the early days and couldn't get her to sleep, or even stop screaming, we would dance to *Metals* by Leslie Feist. "Get It Wrong, Get It Right," the last track on that record, will play when Julie and I are in Puerto Rico or Savannah or somewhere in fifty years and renew our vows.

Here are the songs Feist picked for your marathon:

J.J. Fad, "Supersonic"
Sinéad O'Connor, "Mandinka"
N*E*R*D, "Things Are Getting Better"
Suicide, "Ghost Rider"
Sloan, "She Says What She Means"

25%
INSANE

THE TRAINING: Holy Shit, You're Almost Through!

WEEK 50: Two weeks out from your marathon, try 3 runs. One run should be an easy 8 or 10K (5 or 6 miles). The other should be 10K with 3K (1.9 miles) at race pace—the speed you plan on running in your marathon. Finally, do one last easy 6, 7, or 8K (4 to 5 miles).

WEEK 51: Twice run 5 to 7K (3 to 4.3 miles) super easy, and, 2 days before the race, run an easy 3 to 5K, with 2 or 3 strides of 20 seconds each. This will keep your legs in motion (and also burn up some of that nervous energy).

THE SOUNDTRACK: Jack White

THE FINISH LINE: The marathon, now just about 3 weeks away!

THREE WEEKS AWAY from the marathon, don't run any farther than 10K (6.2 miles). You can't turn yourself into a marathon runner in a week and, at this point, rest is more important than any one run. Run a bit, just to feel tuned up and lean, to keep your legs in motion, and to burn up some overflowing adrenaline. Two weeks out, run three times: do another easy 8 or 10K, and then run something similar a few days later and mix in 3K (1.9 miles) at your race pace. It's cool when you can get a sense of the speed you want to run for the marathon without having to glance at your watch. Again, this is the speed that you think you can maintain across 42.2K (26.2 miles).

When the marathon's seven days away, try to get another three runs in, but all short and easy—5 to 7K (3 to 4.3 miles)—except for working in a few strides. Strides are just little bursts of speed for no more than about twenty seconds, which will get your heart rate up and the blood flowing in your legs. They make you feel fast and ready to race and remind you that you can move quickly. Two days away from your marathon, run 5K with three strides. A day before the big race, watch *Scarface*, call your mother, and cut your toenails.

RUNNING YOUR first marathon is the moment to be brave. You'll be in good company. "It's like you're with all these people who are so much like you, you all have the same personal mission, and we're all like these little warriors," says Tammy Mercier, a runner from Halifax, Nova Scotia, who, like me, will be competing in Boston in three weeks. She says, "Even after sixty-four marathons, I'll stand at the starting line, hear that gun go off and go, 'Shit, this is another twenty-six miles,' but then I start running and I go into a different zone."

Six years ago, Mercier ran her first Boston Marathon, and that morning, as she was lying in bed with her four-year-old, she received a phone call with the news that her father had died. "My daughter said, 'Mommy, are you still going to run?' I said, 'Yes, because Granddaddy taught me how.'" Today,

Mercier has a picture over her desk of her running at Mile 20 at the Boston Marathon on the day her father passed away. She says, "It's to remind me that no matter how tough life gets, if I can get through that, I can get through freaking anything."

Bennett Beach has run forty-five straight Boston Marathons. A father of three based in Bethesda, Maryland, he ran his first Boston at age eighteen in 1968. "It seemed so over the top, so bizarre, that I said, 'I have to do that,'" says Beach, who had steak for breakfast the morning of his first Boston run. "I heard my name announced when approaching the finish line, and it was sort of a fantasy moment for a guy who was never an athlete."

Ten years ago, Beach was diagnosed with dystonia, a neurological problem affecting the brain's synapses and communication with the muscles. He began to limp and injured his hamstring. His running routine dropped to fifteen miles a week, and still he never missed the Boston Marathon. "If you watched me run, you'd say there's no way this guy can finish a marathon, but I just keep stubbornly pushing ahead," says Beach, who was joined by his children, all daughters, forming their own relay team alongside their father on his first race after being diagnosed with the disease. "The sensible reaction to dystonia for a runner is to find another activity—I can ride a bike without a problem—but I can't let go of the marathon. It's probably because I've been doing it so long."

People have different ways of preparing for race day. Reid Coolsaet gets focused, Ryan Hall quotes scripture, Kathrine Switzer thinks of the marathon as a celebration, and Wesley Korir writes his little girl's name on the water bottles he spreads through the course. Matt Loiselle says that all of them, all of us, need to also go 25 percent insane.

"I wouldn't say I have the most talent, but I'm able to bring it when everything's on the line," says Loiselle, who competes in races at every distance from 10K to the marathon and who was preparing for the Vancouver Sun Run when we spoke. There will be almost fifty thousand people running with Loiselle in Vancouver, but for him, the experience is different from that of many of those runners. Loiselle enters races to win. "I know people run the marathon and give a high-five to their family and that's cool—when I do Boston when I'm older, I'll probably do that. I'll stop and grab a beer at the college. But I train 350 days a year for my ten or so races, and I don't want to waste it," he says. "Even when my body's shutting down, I run as hard as I can."

That's the beauty of the marathon and why it's a singular experience: you will be tested. You've trained, you're prepared, and you're ready. But what will you do when that moment's arrived? "When the gun goes off, it's almost eerie—there's thousands of people—but in those last few seconds, I get focused and settle down because I know the hurt's going to come," Loiselle says. "It's exciting—that's why I do it. It's different from normal life, nerve-racking, painful, but I'm 100 percent alive. Not too many people get to experience that, and I'm thankful. I won't be able to do this forever, and I'm thankful I get to do it right now."

Feeling thankful, being excited—all of these are good mind states to get into for the marathon. I want 3:05. I can taste 3:05. Ryan Hall, on his way to the Olympics last summer, told me that to run the marathon you have to be reckless and careful at the same time. "You have to not be afraid to stick your nose in it and fail. I'm the type of runner that would rather blow up one hundred times in order to hit one breakthrough race than have 101 mediocre runs—you have to have *huevos*," says Hall, who echoes Josphat Nzinga and Dick Beardsley, who both said something to the effect that whenever they drop into race mode, they discover something new in themselves.

You're faster than you think you are.

You can run farther than you think you can.

You're tougher than you let yourself believe.

The marathon's about those discoveries. "I've failed many, many times," Hall continues. "I know what it feels like and know I can handle it and be happy in life. As a result, I have no fear, which makes me excited to step on the starting line and swing for the fences. I love putting it all on the line." For us, that doesn't mean competing for our country or trying to set a world record, but Ryan Hall finishing a marathon in 2:04 requires the same kind of effort it takes the average runner to finish his or her first 26.2-mile race.

Betty Lee ran her first marathon in 2011. "There was more a sense of relief after all the training to finally get it over with," says Lee, whose success going from the couch to the marathon in a year taught me that such a thing could even happen. In a sense, she was the inspiration for this book. Deciding she didn't like her sedentary lifestyle, she chose to make a change and then, with grace and humor, made it all the way through injuries and a Canadian winter to the marathon.

Betty Lee ran 42.2K (26.2 miles) in 4:53:58, a 6:10 pace-per-kilometer (9:55 pace-per-mile) for the first 21K (13.1 miles) and a 7:48 (12:33) pace for the last 21. The goal is to run a negative split—which is to run the last half faster than the first half—but it's not easy to do. Even Kenneth Mungara and Ryan Hall have problems with pacing. I managed a negative split in Jerusalem, but that's because I wasn't racing. When you jog, you can listen to music, talk to a friend, even stop by the dry cleaner and pick up your suit. It's an easy pace, and you can often finish faster than you start. When you run, you're engaged and you're thinking about time goals. You're probably not smiling, and you'll need a couple of minutes to catch your breath before you can change a diaper. Racing, however, is yet another ball game: when you race, afterward you really should only be capable of about twenty-five minutes in a bath. You give everything you've got when you're racing, and sometimes adrenaline can lead you astray. "You get it in your head for some reason on race day that you're just going to wake up and the pain's going to be gone and you're going to run a really great time, and I started off good, I really did," says Lee, who ran smoothly for the first 8K (5 miles) and then began feeling her IT band tighten up. At 12K (7.4 miles), she tried changing her gait. The downhill running had been hurting her feet, which had given her problems throughout her training. "I felt like there was a rock in my shoe and I just kept cursing the pain," says Lee, adding that for her, this is where race day's insanity comes into play. On any other day, under these conditions, she would've hailed a cab and gone home. After all, she wasn't even halfway yet and her body was breaking down.

"You tell yourself whatever you have to, to get through it, but I never thought about quitting. I'm sort of limping along, ebbing forward, and then someone called out, 'Go Betty!' It was enough to get me to the next block," she says. "Then I saw a police cruiser coming toward me, and it was a surreal moment—there was a guy running with him, the guy in first place [Kenneth Mungara]—and it was just him and me. As he ran by, I hooted. That put a smile on my face."

Lee reached the halfway point, and then the race changed. She let go of finishing in any specific time and concentrated instead on completing, and enjoying, the experience (as much as she could on two hurting feet and a tight IT band). "I had to release the idea in my head that I was going to finish with any sort of fast time, and then it was almost like all my senses woke up and I could see things more clearly," says Lee, who then thanked her first volunteer, something she would continue to do through the remaining three hours of her race. She had planned on running for ten minutes and then walking for one but realized she'd need to walk more than that. She accepted that fact and she walked most of the route between 30 and 36K (18.6 and 22.4 miles), and then she picked up her jog.

"A friend told me I smiled at her as I got close to the finish line, but I don't think so. I had no energy left in my face," says Lee. "I threw my hands up with fifty meters left. I was so excited I could barely contain myself. I ran across the finish line." That's 25 percent insane.

THE SOUNDTRACK: Jack White
Everyone should have the great good fortune of visiting Jack White's studio in Nashville at least once. Even if you hate his music—and if you hate The White Stripes, really, I don't know what to say—but his place is so out there, all taxidermy and skeletons, red and white walls and tiles, black towels in the bathroom, a huge elephant carcass behind his weird, enormous solid oak desk... I mean, if the guy weren't a rock star, there'd be a dozen police cars outside his studio every night.

At the height of Jack White's popularity, when The White Stripes became pop radio stars with "Seven Nation Army" off *Elephant* in 2003, he took the band off the road, hunkered down in Nashville, and made a record with Loretta Lynn. Cash clearly wasn't guiding his creative decisions. Success meant he could follow his muse.

Meeting White at his studio in Nashville is like sharing chocolate with Willy Wonka at his factory, and I found him cool, strange, down-to-earth, even funny. A guy I was with on the press trip asked him who he thought his contemporaries were, and he answered, Beck. Now I always ask musicians that question. The great Jack White recommended two songs.

"On the Run," Pink Floyd: "When I was a kid, I used to think that song sounded like someone running. There's footsteps, and you can kind of hear that running rhythm. I think synthesizer music's the way to go to get that pounding."

"Baba O'Riley," The Who: "'Won't Get Fooled Again' is another good one, but 'Baba O'Riley' has that pounding synthesizer, that pounding rhythm, that you just can't do on the drums. It's a whole different rhythm than a drum beat and, when you run, your whole body's moving. That's why people think each step should be a kick drum, but that's not the case. It's faster than that. It's 'Baba O'Riley.' It's triple time."

26

RACE FOUR, RUNNING BLISS: BOSTON

THE IMAGE in my head is of me as an assassin, and I break from the starting line with death in my eyes. It's hot in Boston, 27 degrees (80°F) at Mile 0 at 10 a.m., and this gives me a great advantage: I like the heat. I went to school in Tucson. The sun gives me strength. All I need is to clock my 4:23 race pace, but it's the Boston Marathon and I feel too fast for that.

The run starts out in Hopkinton, which is this quaint little American farm town. Runners mill around on the steps of a church before the starting line, and there's a small-town feel to the calm before the big race. It's as if all 26,000 of us are in the same band, just about to take the stage. The gun goes off, and I'm jetting. It feels good not to be waiting anymore, and I'm kicking hard, pumping my arms with my fingers extended, moving with aerodynamic purpose and a big, beautiful, long stride.

There are no pacers at Boston, and so my plan's to attach myself to another 3:05 runner, but there's not really a convivial vibe among participants. Everyone's here to work, and ultimately, running's something you must do on your own.

I'm out here now in attack mode. Five kilometers come and go like the view of a tourist attraction from inside a car. I hit 5K (3 miles) in 22:25, which is odd—that's thirty seconds slower than where I should be. I grab some water and dump it on my head. I think maybe Tucson's supposed to be a dry heat, and anyway, that was twenty years ago. How do I know how I'll respond to running a marathon on Mars?

The sun feels like a laser beam. I try a bit of reframing: I'm an assassin who's been injured, maybe clipped in the arm, trying, for the sake of his family, to pull off one last job. My kick is good and my head's up. I pass the Ashland Clock Tower and the Framingham Train Station and I'm toeing a true straight line, concentrating not on being deerlike but on being like a cheetah in pursuit of a deer.

I drop 10K (6 miles) in 44:47, almost a full minute behind my race plan, and the disappointment hits me right in the calf. I'm working awfully hard to be failing, a feeling that I'm familiar with, but not usually when I run. The tightness in my calf spreads to my hamstring, and 10K to 11K (6.8 miles) feels like a flight cross-country with a screaming kid. I need to, and can't, escape the sun. I yell. I don't want to give up. I pass some asshole running in bare feet who gets all the cheers from the crowd, which blithely ignores my plight. I keep my back straight. I'm a superhero. I tilt back my head. But it's like my alter ego slowly inhales the kryptonite and now hobbles a little, trying to kick out his leg pain, and I pop an energy gel that doesn't do shit. I speed up. I slow down. One thing I don't do is run 4:23 per kilometer (7:03 per mile), and the split times on my hand might as well be a tattoo I regret that I got in college.

My 15K (9.3 miles) is 1:07:35. I've added another fat minute to my time. My sneakers feel tight; I've only run in them once before. And my shirt feels heavy—choosing a shirt for its pocket was a tactical error—and I'm dying in this unbearable heat. I know that you shouldn't race in something you haven't worn before but here I am, in the Boston Marathon, doing just that. My socks, however, are terrific. Unfortunately, they're not enough.

Forty-two kilometers is a journey, and the Boston Marathon goes from the sticks to Beantown's famous urban core. It's extraordinary how the city's responding. There are helicopters circling above, both news and emergency, and as the hour approaches 11:30, there are more and more college kids lining the course with drinks in hand. I yearn for one of those glasses. Why, I wonder, do I do this again?

Runners congregate at either edge of the course where the aid stations are because water's so important, and I'm dumping as much of it on my head as I swallow. Should I take off my shirt? It's got the bib with my race number pinned to it, and that bib contains the tracking device that's keeping score of my time. Now soaking with sweat and water, my stupid shirt with a zipper must weigh ten kilograms or maybe it just feels that way as I knock through 19K (11.8 miles) at 1:30:48—an ungodly six minutes off my projected time. A whole year of training, for this.

It's here that I come upon a crossroad. My left leg is like a DVD player incorrectly attached to a TV: I cannot get it to function. It's not that I have an injury. It's more like a wire in my circuitry's blown. Around me, I see runners keel over on the sidelines and watch a woman throw up green oatmeal. I'm not leaving this thing in a wheelchair, I decide, and I take a breath.

My pace drops to 4:52, a time I maintain on my easy runs. When I reach Wellesley College just before the halfway mark, the spirit—the animation, the cheering, the history—touches me and I smile. Somewhere, probably somewhere in front of me, Bennett Beach and Tammy Mercier are running proudly, and mentally I cheer them on. It's just not my morning in Boston, and 24K (14.9 miles) into my marathon, I walk. Julie, through parts unknown, pushes Esme in her stroller. Trying to find space in a heat emergency amid 500,000 people. I turn on my music, feeling thankful, and a live version of "Nothing As It Seems" by Pearl Jam takes me almost to ecstasy.

I eat a banana. I play air guitar. I throw an arm up in the air. I'm going to control the experience. I'm in Boston, with my wife and baby, and there are complete strangers cheering me on. Fuck my time.

"You're doing awesome," says someone kind.

"Thank you for being here," I reply.

Eventually, I flounce across the finish line at 3:58:54, a time that should've been ample enough for me to have raced, found Julie and Esme, showered, and begun tracking down the tavern in Boston with the coldest beer. Instead, I sheepishly crawl back to my hotel room and draw a bath. Twenty minutes later, Julie, Esme, and I reunite in the bathroom.

Funny, when I tell them that the Boston Marathon took me nearly four hours, neither of them seems to care.

FOOTNOTES

A YEAR AFTER I finished the Boston Marathon, bombs went off at 2:49 p.m., four hours, nine minutes, and forty-three seconds after the race began, and at least 264 people were injured and three people were killed. There are things that you can't control in a marathon, and things that should never be.

Congratulations on your race, however you did, and thank you for spending fifty-two weeks with me on the run. What you did, however you did, is an accomplishment—don't ever forget that. And I hope that your journey's not done. But when you're running, think about the people who lost their lives in Boston, all the victims and their families. Never forget how lucky you are. When running, remember that you're fortunate to have your health, to have the time and resources to pursue your hobby. Even though running makes you healthier, happier, and, I'd argue, more sane, a hobby is still all it is. Don't get lost in your training. Like Julie said, put the dickhead away. To reach the marathon takes dedication, aching muscles, lots of laundry, cool bosses, setbacks, and pain. I wish you luck, encouragement, faith, motivation, and a big tub of petroleum jelly in your pursuit.

So take a week after your marathon and forget running. Load up on veal parmesan and ice-cold martinis and all the things you denied yourself for too long. Mow the lawn and take your wife or husband dancing. Above everything, when your race is finished, I hope, eventually, you'll be looking forward to racing again. I can't wait to see you out at an event.

Me? I'd have liked to come in about an hour faster, but what are you going to do? At this point, it's all just kilometers under my shoes. Anyway, now it's Julie's turn to get cracking. The former volleyball star's signed up for her first 5 K with her mother. I offered to pace them, but, go figure, they signed up for a women's only run.

When you put labels in front of your name, what words do you use? I can think of a long string of words, things I've been and will likely continue to be, but I prefer this one: runner. And now you're a runner, too. By this point, you've probably experienced enough ups and downs with the sport, enough chafed nipples and sore feet and perhaps even worse, to last a lifetime. But no one knows the extent of their capabilities. We may never walk on the moon or stand up to a tank in the name of freedom. However, every one of us gets the opportunity every day, every hour, to be our loved one's hero. I think about that sometimes when I'm running, pushing myself. We can be better. We can do more. We can find the strength to keep going. In the end, that's all running's about. Godspeed.

THE SOUNDTRACK: Ben Kaplan
Every person in the book—every athlete, every coach, every celebrity, every runner—is a hero of mine, someone I think's worth listening to. I can vouch for all of the bands that've recommended music. There were a lot of other musicians I cornered who gave me songs that, eventually, I decided I had to

cut out: all of these performers—even Justin Bieber and Selena Gomez—have chops. They wouldn't be in here if I didn't think they were good. So here are their greatest running songs, as picked out by me.

The Black Eyed Peas, "Let's Get Retarded": There was a time when men would make other men mixed tapes and include the music of The Black Eyed Peas. For me, this song, the original, which would change the way will.i.am wrote music, is their battle cry.

Paul Simon, "Graceland": For the lyrics, for the groove, for the tempo, this is the best song on an unbelievably good record, with a double-time beat that threatens to carry you out of your shoes. "The Boxer" also is really, really good.

Justin Bieber, "Maria": Bieber's got a dark side, and in this last song on *Believe*, he swings back at the woman who accused him of fathering her kid. Bieber's grown up? On this track he is. You can tell he's been hanging with Usher.

Ghostface Killah, "Run": Make sure you get the remix with Jadakiss. "I might gotta take my shirt off," he says, before starting his rap. When he's finished, you might have to, too.

Broken Social Scene, "Almost Crimes" and "Anthems for a Seventeen Year Old Girl": The first one features Feist and the second has Metric's Emily Haines, and I can't pick just one. You can't make me.

Kendrick Lamar, "The Art of Peer Pressure": That a day in the life of a Compton teenager sounds exactly relatable to a bald middle-aged Jewish father in Canada speaks to the universality of Mr. Lamar. That he has hip hop's best flow doesn't hurt either.

Carrie Underwood, "Before He Cheats": This is a pop rock new country story revenge song, but I guess I lied, sorta. I don't really know Carrie Underwood's music at all.

Death Cab for Cutie/The Postal Service, "Such Great Heights": It's important to switch tempos on a long running mixed tape; you don't want your music to pound, pound, pound song after song. "Such Great Heights" is dreamy and soaring—makes you feel like you can fly.

Lionel Richie, "Hello": I'll run to a ballad. Why can't I? Nostalgia, more than beats-per-minute, gets me up difficult hills.

Dolly Parton, "Jolene": Short and feisty and barbed like the wire on the outside of a jail, this punchy little number turns open hands into fists. If you like this song, there's a version out there that Jack White does, too.

Marilyn Manson, "The Dope Show": Expect the monster chorus to hit you like 59 Red Bulls. For such a visual artist, Manson's actually better when you don't have to look at his pants.

Michael Bublé, "Home": So what? I LIKE getting emotional when I run. I also listen to Snow Patrol and Neil Diamond.

Guns N' Roses, "Paradise City": The reason I started writing about music—and when was the last time you threw it on? It still sounds just as awesome. And remember, it's OK to rewind.

Brian Wilson, "God Only Knows": All this time out there on your own, in your own little world, it's nice to think about the person you love.

Metric, "Combat Baby": *No one here wants to fight me like you do.* Perhaps it's the perfect song: punky, poppy, and jagged. Like bubblegum tequila. Short too.

Willie Nelson, "On the Road Again": It's hard to listen to this and not smile. I love the words and the message. Plus, Willie Nelson's a runner, who knew?

Joan Baez, "Diamonds and Rust": Soul over speed metal any day.

Moby, "South Side": The version with Gwen Stefani almost makes me want to spread out my arms like a plane. I've interviewed Moby twenty-five times. Twenty-five times I've learned something new.

The Cranberries, "Zombie": Really? You don't like this song? Are you nuts?

The National, "Bloodbuzz, Ohio": One hundred-and-fifty-seven beats per minute. These guys aren't my favourite. But Julie prefers them to G'N'R.

The Gaslight Anthem, "American Slang": Even though I live in Toronto, a man's DNA doesn't change.

Young Jeezy, "Put On" (featuring Jay-Z): It's hard to have stooped posture when this song's bumping—a declaration to hometown pride with one of my all-time favorite verses from Jay-Z.

Katy Perry, "Hot n Cold": Remember, there's no penalty for singing out loud.

The Black Keys, "Gold on the Ceiling": The freakin' guitars are like hacksaws! For whatever reason, I've always felt like this one had a Blues Brothers vibe. They'd like that, I bet.

Pearl Jam, "Nothing As It Seems": Get the live version. Saved my life.

Norah Jones, "Miriam": It's fun to listen to what happens when Norah Jones gets her gun. *Miriam/That's such a pretty name/I'm gonna say it when I make you cry.* It doesn't hurt that Danger Mouse, the guy who made this record, also did "Crazy" by Gnarls Barkley.

Feist, "Graveyard": If you had to give up alcohol, coffee, or music, what would it be? Definitely coffee, OK. But then what? Sometimes, I get tempted to say music. Then I play this song.

Jack White, "I Just Don't Know What To Do With Myself": The crunch at the end of this White Stripes' track will probably take at least three seconds off your marathon time. At the very least, it always makes me want to get back on the road.

Enjoy.

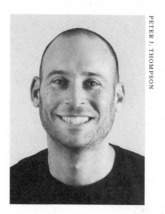

BEN KAPLAN writes about running and music for the *National Post* and is a co-founder of EachCoach.com. His work has appeared in *GQ*, *New York* magazine, *Cosmopolitan*, and the *New York Times*. He lives in Toronto with his wife and baby daughter.